AF544830

JAN VAN RYMSDYK

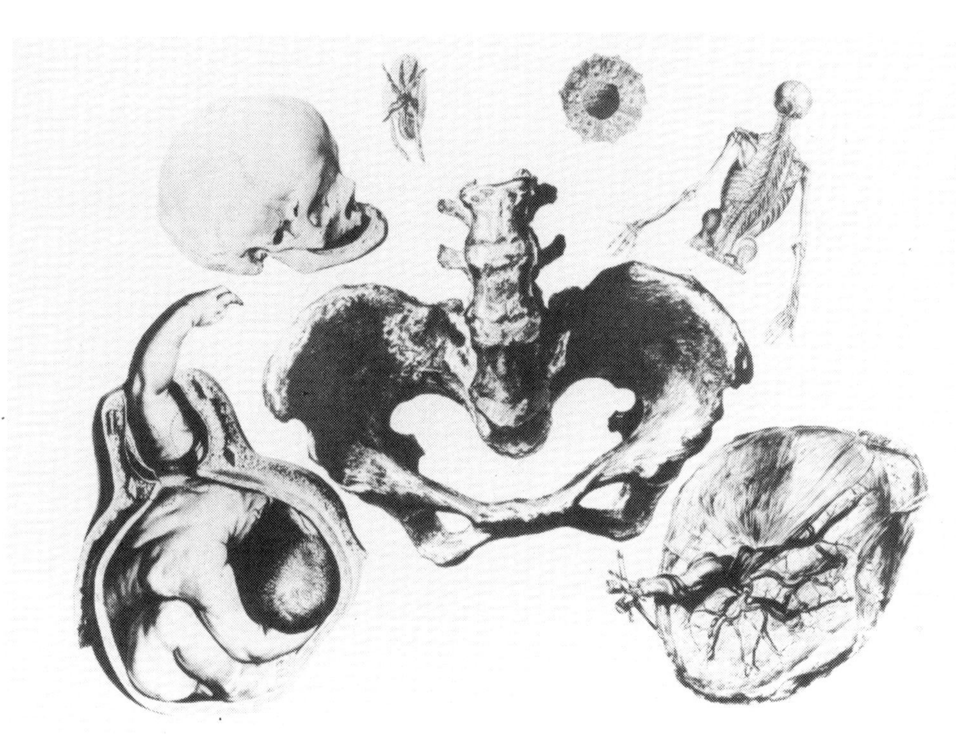

JAN VAN RYMSDYK

Medical Artist of the Eighteenth Century

by

JOHN L. THORNTON F.L.A.

Formerly Librarian
St. Bartholomew's Hospital Medical College
and Consultant Librarian
Royal College of Obstetricians and Gynaecologists

The OLEANDER Press
Cambridge · New York

The Oleander Press
17 Stansgate Avenue
Cambridge CB2 2QZ
England

The Oleander Press
210 Fifth Avenue
New York
N.Y. 10010
U.S.A.

First published 1982

British Library Cataloguing in Publication Data

Thornton, John Leonard
Jan Van Rymsdyk
1. Medical illustration - Biography
I. Title
610' .28 R836

ISBN 0-906672-02-3

Typeset and printed in Great Britain.

CONTENTS

Preface

List of Illustrations

Chapter 1 Jan Van Rymsdyk 1

Chapter 2 Rymsdyk's drawings for William Smellie (1697-1763) 10

Chapter 3 Rymsdyk's drawings for William Hunter (1718-1783) 22

Chapter 4 Rymsdyk's drawings for John Hunter (1728-1793) 43

Chapter 5 Rymsdyk's drawings for Charles Nicholas Jenty 53

Chapter 6 The *Museum Britannicum* 61

Chapter 7 Andrew Van Rymsdyk (1753 or 1754-1786) 75

Chapter 8 Rymsdyk's drawings for Thomas Denman (1733-1815), and others 82

Chapter 9 Rymsdyk's influence on medical book illustration 89

Bibliography 94

Index 100

PREFACE

Illustrations in medical books are often of greater importance than the text, and this is particularly true of the older textbooks. Written to instruct both students and established members of the profession, the plates elucidate the text, and can convey to viewers at a glance more information than can be gleaned from laboriously poring over many pages of manuscript or printed text. Furthermore, they are international, and can be comprehended without translation, by readers throughout the world. In antique books, their value has usually outlasted that of the texts they illustrate, and many anatomical atlases owe their current interest to the beauty and accuracy of their plates.

Seldom have the artists responsible for the original drawings received adequate recognition for their work, and this book is an attempt to remedy this by salvaging the scanty relics of the life and work of the outstanding medical artist of the eighteenth century, Jan Van Rymsdyk. His name is sometimes linked with those for whom he worked, but little is known of his life, despite research extending over many years. This book is an attempt to consolidate the information gained, and to provide specimens of his work, which may inspire other medical artists in the pursuit of their profession.

During the years that have elapsed since I first became interested in Jan Van Rymsdyk I have been in contact with many people who have assisted me in my research. Without attempting to name all of them, I must mention the following for providing information, photographs and encouragement:

Dr. John Huffman, of Michigan, who initially wrote two articles on Rymsdyk after extensive research, but was forced by ill-health to abandon the task, and encouraged me to continue the study: Dr. Helen Brock, Research Fellow in the Department of the History of Science at Glasgow University, and Mr. Jack Baldwin, Keeper of the Special Collections in the University Library, both of whom have greatly assisted me with information on the Rymsdyk drawings in the Hunterian Collection; Mr. William R. LeFanu, formerly

Librarian, Mr. Eustace Cornelius, Librarian, and Mr. Ian Lyle, of the Royal College of Surgeons of England; Mr. Anthony J. Beeson, Fine Art Librarian, Avon County Library, Bristol, Miss Judith Dyer, Hospital Librarian, Bristol Royal Infirmary, Mr. F. W. Greenacre, Curator of Fine Art, Bristol Museum and Art Gallery, and Miss Mary E. Williams, the City Archivist; Mr. F. J. Hill, Department of Printed Books, and Mr. John Gorton, Department of Manuscripts, British Library, and Mr. Reginald Williams, Department of Prints and Drawings, British Museum; Mr. D. G. C. Allan, Curator-Librarian, Royal Society of Arts; The Victoria and Albert Museum, London; the National Gallery of Ireland, Dublin; Birmingham City Library; Dr. John B. Blake, History of Medicine Division, National Library of Medicine, Washington; Mrs. Caroline Morris, Librarian-Archivist, Pennsylvania Hospital; Dr. An Zwollo, Rijksbureau voor Kunsthistorische Documentatie, The Hague; Professor William S. Heckscher, Princeton University Library; Miss Antonia J. Bunch, Miss Jessie Dobson, Miss Ruth Gilmour, Mrs. Janet Bower, Mary Countess of Pembroke, and Miss Gertrude Hill. In addition to the libraries named above, I have made extensive use of those at the Royal College of Obstetricians and Gynaecologists, where Miss Patricia C. Want and Miss Mary Evans have been most helpful; the Wellcome Historical Medical Library; and St. Bartholomew's Hospital Medical College. Miss Carole Reeves has provided some of the photographs, and Mrs. Ann Munson has typed the numerous versions of the manuscript.

Finally, I must thank the Leverhulme Trust Fund for the award of a Leverhulme Emeritus Fellowship (1979–81), which has contributed significantly towards the acquisition of photographs of most of Rymsdyk's original drawings and paintings, and has enabled me to complete this study more effectively than would have been possible without that assistance. The photographs and other material will be deposited in the Royal College of Obstetricians and Gynaecologists Library.

Wembley, June 1981 John L. Thornton

LIST OF ILLUSTRATIONS

		page
Plate 1	Jan Van Rymsdyk's portrait of William Barrett, painted in 1764. (City of Bristol Museum and Art Gallery).	8
Plate 2	Engraving by Charles Grignion of Jan Van Rymsdyk's portrait of William Smellie, painted or drawn in 1753. (By permission of the Harveian Librarian, Royal College of Physicians of London).	13
Plate 3	Rymsdyk's original drawing of the gravid uterus in the eighth or ninth month of pregnancy. Engraved as Table 9 in Smellie's *Sett of anatomical tables,* 1754. (Hunterian Collection, University of Glasgow).	18
Plate 4	Rymsdyk's original drawing of Smellie's forceps in position around head of fetus. Engraved as Table 21 in Smellie's *Sett of anatomical tables,* 1754. (Hunterian Collection, University of Glasgow).	19
Plate 5	Title-page of William Hunter's *Gravid uterus,* 1774.	28
Plate 6	Rymsdyk's original drawing, dated 1750, of the fetus at term in the womb, for William Hunter's *Gravid uterus,* 1774. (Hunterian Collection, University of Glasgow).	33
Plate 7	Engraving by Robert Strange of Rymsdyk's original drawing for William Hunter's *Gravid uterus,* 1774, Table VI.	34
Plate 8	Rymsdyk's original drawing of retroverted womb in fifth month of pregnancy, for William Hunter's *Gravid uterus,* 1774, Table XXVI, Figure 1. The book and lower limbs are not	36

featured in the engraving. (Hunterian Collection, University of Glasgow).

Plate 9 Rymsdyk's original drawing of a fully opened womb containing a fetus at the beginning of the fifth month of pregnancy, for William Hunter's *Gravid uterus,* 1774. This was engraved as Table XXVII, Figure II. (Hunterian Collection, University of Glasgow). 37

Plate 10 Rymsdyk's original drawing of skull for Plate III, Figure 2 of John Hunter's *Natural history of the human teeth,* 1771. The lower half only was engraved, and the initials on the end of the book were omitted. (By permission of the President and Council of the Royal College of Surgeons of England). 46

Plate 11 Rymsdyk's original drawings for Plate IV, Figures 1 and 2 of John Hunter's *Natural history of the human teeth,* 1771. Only the upper half of the top figure was engraved. (By permission of the President and Council of the Royal College of Surgeons of England). 47

Plates 12–13 Series of drawings by Rymsdyk showing the development of the chick. These are in colour, and the two framed pictures hang in the Hunterian Museum. (By permission of the President and Council of the Royal College of Surgeons of England). 50 51

Plate 14 Mezzotint version of Rymsdyk's coloured drawing for C. N. Jenty's *Demonstration of the human structure,* 1757, Table 1. 56

Plate 15 Mezzotint of Rymsdyk's drawings of the pregnant uterus at term, from C. N. Jenty's *Demonstrations of a pregnant uterus,* 1757, Table 4. 59

Plates –17 Title-pages of the two editions of *Museum Britannicum* by Jan and Andrew Van Rymsdyk, 1778 and 1791. (Wellcome Institute for the History of Medicine). 63 68

Plates 18–19 Original drawings for Plates V and VI of *Museum Britannicum* Plate V is by Jan, and Plate VI is by Andrew Van Rymsdyk. (By permission of the Trustees of the British Museum). 71 72

Plate 20 Engraved version of Jan Van Rymsdyk's drawing of the gravid uterus at term, from Thomas Denman's *Collection of engravings,* 1787. 86

1

JAN VAN RYMSDYK

"The world knows nothing of its greatest men."
Henry Taylor.

Despite the fact that his name is well known to medical historians as the artist responsible for the remarkable drawings in the atlases of William Smellie and William Hunter, very little is known about Jan Van Rymsdyk's life. Standard reference books provide very little information, and most of this is inaccurate. John W. Huffman (1969 and 1970) spent some time in Leyden trying to trace Rymsdyk's ancestry and his activities before he came to London, but with no success, and we were left with his illustrations as almost the only evidence of his existence. Huffman's two papers, in which he recorded the work of Rymsdyk known at that time, were intended as preliminary studies, but unfortunately the author was unable to pursue his research. The present book summarises the results of further investigation.

The spelling of his name varies on the engraved versions of his drawings, the lettering being added later, but when he signed them, he used "Jan Van Rymsdyk", "J. V. Rymsdyk", or the initials "J. V. R." We find him mentioned as Riemsdyk, Rijmsdyk, Reimsdyk, Remsdyk, and often with a final "e" added. On the title page of his *Museum Britannicum* we find "John" rather than "Jan", but this appears to be a rare occasion. His son Andreas, however, adopted "Andrew" early in life, and later advertised himself simply as "Andrew Rymsdyk".

Despite intensive searching, and the co-operation of various genealogical sources, we have been unable to trace where and when Jan Van Rymsdyk was born. He was certainly born in Holland, and in the *Museum Britannicum* (see Chapter 6) he gives proof of this on several occasions, e.g. "witness my Country, the Republic of Holland", (p. 26), and, "For Mr. Lewenhoek (Leeuwenhoek), my Countryman, (*etc.*), (p. 38, footnote). Writing not later than 1776 he also states:

> "And I remember once about thirty-six years ago, in a walk from the Hague to Scheveling, I met with an old Dutch Sailor, who was then a Fisherman;" (*etc.*) (p. 41, footnote).

This was probably about 1740, and suggests that Rymsdyk was no longer a child at that time. He again mentions the "famous Village the Hague", (p. 78, footnote), and also a Dutch physician at The Hague using his hands to communicate with the dumb, (p. 71, footnote). Rymsdyk also mentions being in Amsterdam, when writing on asbestos:

> "Cloth as well as paper has been made of this Stone, and I have seen a Gentleman, a kind of Philosopher, at Amsterdam, who had a tasty Night-cap of it, which when foul he would throw it into the fire, and became better clean than if it had been washed with soap and water, as we do linen", (p. 55, footnote).

Also in *Museum Britannicum,* Rymsdyk mentions his father on two occasions. After discussing the dangers of using white copper in making culinary or kitchen furniture he continues:

> "I am obliged to my Father for the above information, otherwise I should have engaged in Partnership with a Copper-Smith many years ago," (p. 21); and again, "My Father, in 1757, had a large white Hen, which frequently used to lay Eggs with two yolks in each", (p. 17).

This suggests the possibility that Jan Van Rymsdyk's father came to England with him, and was certainly alive and in contact with Jan seven years after the latter arrived in London.

Rymsdyk appeared in London in 1750, and it has been suggested that he came there from Bristol, but we have no concrete evidence that he was in that city until 1758. The only possible evidence of his having been there before then was the fact that a portrait of Thomas Page, Surgeon to Bristol Royal Infirmary at the time of his death on 5 May 1741, was attributed to Rymsdyk, although it is not signed or dated. We examined the manuscript Richard Smith's "Bristol Infirmary Biographical Memoirs, 1735–77", volume two of which contains pencilled drawings of several portraits, including that of Thomas Page. Opposite this (on page 111) is the following note:

> "The portrait of Mr. Thomas Page, probably by Fry – was given to me by Mrs. Martha Sprague (added in margin, "in 1824") – widow of the Rev'd. Daniel Sprague, but it was to remain with her until her decease – which happened about April 1831. I placed it against the wall in my Museum at the Infirmary. Fry is mentioned by Boswell in his life of Johnson Page 4, Vol. 2d in a footnote".

This was probably Thomas Frye (1710–1762), the painter and engraver, who also discovered the method of making porcelain. He occupied himself with this for fifteen years in Bow, before resuming his original profession. This suggests that the attribution of the portrait of Thomas Page to Rymsdyk was erroneous, and leaves no grounds for supposing that the was in Bristol before the death of Thomas Page in 1741.

London in the eighteenth century was experiencing an age of transition. Following the Plague of 1665 and the Great Fire of 1666 there had been extensive replanning of the City itself, and much rebuilding had taken place. Priority was given to municipal buildings, premises for merchants and business men, followed by numerous churches, and the main roads were ribboned by frontages of newly erected edifices. The streets were still narrow, as were the frontages, the premises extending to the rear with gardens, stables and similar erections. Behind the main thoroughfares were the courts, alleys and lanes for shopkeepers, artisans and others necessary to staff the business interests of the City. Many of the survivors from the pestilence and fire did not return, but settled in the surrounding districts. Sanitation was still lacking, and the death rate among children in particular remained high. This persisted until about 1750, when William Smellie and others provided better education for midwives, and improved medical services were made available by the foundation of new hospitals, the rebuilding of others, and the opening of dispensaries for those unable to afford the high fees of the physicians. Some of these gave their services free by staffing these dispensaries, and were also able to assist patients to gain admittance to hospital if necessary.

It is apparent that progress in building and in the improvement of social conditions was not continuous. In fact, the century saw progression in waves of prosperity and periods of regression, caused by wars on the Continent and in America, and unsettled times at home. The first half of the century saw the continuation of building, with the erection of many houses outside the City bounds, and those engaged in the various building trades prospered, architects, stonemasons, bricklayers and carpenters in particular being in demand. Sir John Summerson (1978) has provided an excellent illustrated account of Georgian London, and M. Dorothy George (1979) has written a well-documented survey of social conditions in eighteenth century London. The previous century has been called "the age of scientific endeavour", but the great figures of that period were not readily replaced by others capable of sustaining the search for medical and scientific knowledge. In fact, the first half of the eighteenth century saw the publication of very few outstanding medical books in England, and the writings of William Cheselden (1688–1752) stand almost alone as outstanding medical publications from London during that fifty years.

The lack of sanitation still resulted in epidemics, and the availability of cheap gin resulted in drunkenness and crime among the poorer classes. Class distinction was evident at several levels, and was particularly recognisable in houses where the poorest were lodged in basements and garrets, with those of higher social standing on their respective floors between. Overcrowding was evident by more than one family occupying small rooms, and by many persons sleeping on the floor of others. Criminals infested the back streets and alleys, and it was unsafe to venture out in the dark. There were many migrants from provincial towns and the surrounding countryside, and immigrants from Ireland and France, the latter in particular settling in particular areas. There were also Jews from Holland and Germany. Some of them brought with them skills in arts and crafts, and established new industries. Many were attracted by rumours of "streets paved with gold", as in succeeding centuries, but most quickly became disillusioned. Then, as now, the rich generally increased their wealth, and the poor gradually sank deeper into poverty, frustrated by lack of work, low wages, high prices, and poor housing. In the middle of the eighteenth century there was an improvement, and steps began to be taken towards the betterment of sanitation, health, the care of the sick, child welfare, and education in general, but it was only the beginning of a very slow process. In fact, it is still in progress.

This was London when we first find Rymsdyk working there. It was probably no worse than any other large town in England, and no better, but it did appear to offer opportunities for those with skills to offer. Jan Van Rymsdyk was certainly in London in 1750, when we know he was making drawings for William Hunter (see Chapter 2), but we know little of his career before that date. He was obviously a brilliant artist, and it has been suggested that he must have been conversant with anatomical material and techniques before commencing work with Hunter. However, no original drawings or illustrations by him have been traced before that date, and speculation has been the sole source of these suggestions. We do not know Rymsdyk's age at that time, but his son Andrew (Andreas) was born in either 1753 or 1754 (see Chapter 7). We also know nothing about this wife, but assume that he was married, and do not know where he was living. It is possible that he lived in the Hunter household, as it was usual to have staff living on the premises, and we know that John Hunter, at a later date, had artists, printers and others residing at his homes both in London and Earl's Court.

Rymsdyk started drawing the first ten plates for William Hunter's *Gravid uterus* in 1750, and continued at intervals until 1772, when he made the fourth drawing on Plate 34 (see Chapter 3). The book was finally published in 1774, twenty-four years after the first drawing was executed. William Smellie's *Anatomical tables* was published in 1754, but Rymsdyk had completed the drawings for twenty-two of the illustrations by 1752, so that he was obviously working simultaneously for Smellie and Hunter. He also painted or drew a portrait of Smellie in 1753, but the original version has not been traced (see Chapter 2).

In 1755 Rymsdyk was also making drawings for Charles Nicholas Jenty (see Chapter 5), whose *Essay on the demonstration of the human structure,* with four plates, and *Demonstrations of a pregnant uterus,* with six plates, were published in 1757. In addition he was working for John Hunter, who was assisting William Hunter in his anatomy school. Many of these drawings for John Hunter were not published for many years; in fact, some for *The natural history of the human teeth,* published in 1771, were probably drawn "before the year 1755" (see Chapter 4). These activities must have kept Rymsdyk fully occupied after his arrival in London in 1750, but apparently he was unhappy with his work as a medical artist. Possibly he could no longer tolerate the conditions pervading the atmosphere of dissecting rooms, with corpses of both humans and animals cut open for him to depict on paper. He fancied himself as a portrait painter, but the only record of his activity in this field at that time which we know is that of William Smellie. Following that, Rymsdyk might have expected further commissions through the influence of William Hunter, but these were not forthcoming.

We know that in 1758 and 1759 Jan Van Rymsdyk was resident in All Saints Lane, Bristol, and was advertising himself as a portrait painter. Why he went to Bristol we can only speculate upon (unless he had previously been there), but he was obviously dissatisfied with London as the centre of his activities. Bristol already had a long distinguished history by the middle of the eighteenth century, and was second only to London as a centre for trade and commerce. A major port, having an extensive trade with Africa, America and the West Indies, even before the advent of the railway in the next century it had an extensive communication system with all the major towns in the country, both by sea, and by carrier and stage coach. As a centre of the slave trade, and importer of raw materials from abroad, it developed into a large industrial centre with sugar refineries, glass-making factories, and businesses based on chocolate, cotton, tobacco, porcelain, metals and other commodities. No wheeled vehicles were allowed on the narrow cobbled streets, which covered extensive cellars, and traffic was limited to horse-drawn sledges and pack-horses. The city was prosperous, and the rich merchants and businessmen generally lived on their premises, while Bath and Cheltenham were within easy reach. Bristol also had Hotwell, another fashionable spa, only a mile from the city, which attracted famous literary figures, actors, artists and others desirous of obtaining patronage from the wealthy. A comprehensive introductory history of the area has been written by Brian S. Smith and Elizabeth Ralph (1972) in a compact volume which includes numerous maps and other illustrations showing the various aspects of city life through the ages.

This environment might well have attracted Rymsdyk as an alternative to London, and to have offered clientele who might commission him as a portrait painter. He advertised his services in the press, and *Felix Farley's Bristol Journal* for 13 January 1759 carried the following advertisement:

> "J. V. Riemsdyk, portrait painter, at his rooms at the Register-Office in All-Saints Lane, Bristol, paints portraits at four guineas each: half lengths, and whole lengths, in proportion. N. B. He instructs gentlemen and ladies in the art of drawing in its several branches, on reasonable terms: – being likewise well known for his drawings of anatomy, herbs, fossils, &c. to the most eminent of the faculty in London. His paintings may be seen any time of the day at his lodgings."

We know that Rymsdyk painted portraits of Thomas Newton (1704–1782), Bishop of Bristol, the original of which is in the City of Bristol Museum and Art Gallery, and of John Page (died 1792), which is in Bristol Royal Infirmary, but neither is signed or dated. In 1762 he painted Dr. Edward Lyne (died 1772), a fact mentioned in Richard Smith's "Biographical memoirs" (vol. 2, pp. 402 and 404), with a pencil copy of the portrait (between pp. 401–2), and an annotation:

> "This was pencilled by Mr. Henry (Gold – ger?) Surgeon 25 Kings Square A.D. 1824 – from the original by J. C. (sic) Rymsdyke S.D. 1762 – the original is in the possession of Mr. Wm. Tyson the bookseller 21 Clare St. – I showed the picture to Mr. Charleton (gentman?) who well remembered (him) & he said it is very like him."

The portrait was reproduced by G. Munro Smith (1917).

Another interesting item appears in Richard Smith's "Biographical memoirs", (p. 202), at the end of a memoir of John Page (volume two, pp. 190–202), with a drawing of him (between 284 and 286):

> "The Painting from which Mr. Smith copied the pencilled drawing prefixed was executed by one Rymsdyke an acquaintance of Old Michael Edkins the painter many years employed in the scenery of the Bristol Theatre & a resident of Bridge Street.
>
> Rymsdyk was a very clever artist, so miserably poor that he was glad to wear the cast off clothes of Mr. Wm. Barrat the Surgeon and Bristol historian. There is an excellent likeness of his painting of Old Allen the organist of Redcliffe nicknamed "Thumbs" – into which he said playing upon that instrument had turned his fingers."

Further to this, a footnote in G. Munro Smith (1917) suggests that Rymsdyk was:

> "according to Mr. William Edkins, 'a tall raw-boned German and excessively proud, although a sign painter'. He was brought into notice, according to Richard Smith, by a sign-board he painted for a public house at the corner of Cart Lane, Temple Street. This was 'Bacchus astride on a tun', and was much admired. He was lazy and generally in need of money, often wearing, according to Mr. Edkins, William Barrett's cast-off clothing."

Later, in his book, G. Munro Smith (1917, p. 226) records the various taverns in Bristol, and again mentions Rymsdyk:

> "The 'Ship' was frequented by musicians, artists and interesting Bohemians, who led a jovial rollicking life. Amongst these characters were Rymsdyke, the painter, who dressed 'in large flap waistcoat, immense cuffs to his coat sleeves, with breeches just to the knee, and slit before, with knee buttons'. Michael Edkins, player and scene painter at the theatre, Jem Sewell, afterwards landlord of the Talbot Tavern in Redcliff Street, Joe Gillard the rope-maker, "Thumb" Allen and others. These good fellows used to meet at the 'Ship', then under the care of 'Landlord' Wyat, and drink the beer for which the inn was famous."

A pencil portrait of William Barrett (1733–1789) mentioned above, is also included in Richard Smith's *Biographical memoirs* (volume two, between pp. 284 and 286) with a biographical memoir of him (pp. 286–295). He practised mainly as a surgeon and "man midwife", and wrote a history of Bristol; the original portrait is in Bristol Museum and Art Gallery, having been purchased in 1954 from Miss Karina Maas. This portrait, painted by Rymsdyk in 1764, was engraved by William Walker, and published by William Strong, "bookseller, Bristol & Exeter". The engraving is an abbreviated version of the original, which includes a finely executed hand with a lace cuff, holding a skull resting on a book (Plate 1).

From existing evidence we must conclude that Jan Van Rymsdyk's sojourn in Bristol was not a success; he appears to have painted few portraits, and was forced to paint inn signs, and to wear the cast-off clothes of William Barrett. We do not know if he took his wife (if indeed he had one), and Andrew with him, but he seems to have spent much of his time in taverns in the company of those leading "a jovial, rollicking life." In 1764 Andrew reached ten years of age, and Jan Van Rymsdyk painted the portrait of William Barrett, possibly his last. In that year he returned to London, probably as disillusioned about portrait painting in Bristol as he had been in London.

Both John Hunter and Charles Nicholas Jenty had joined the Army, and

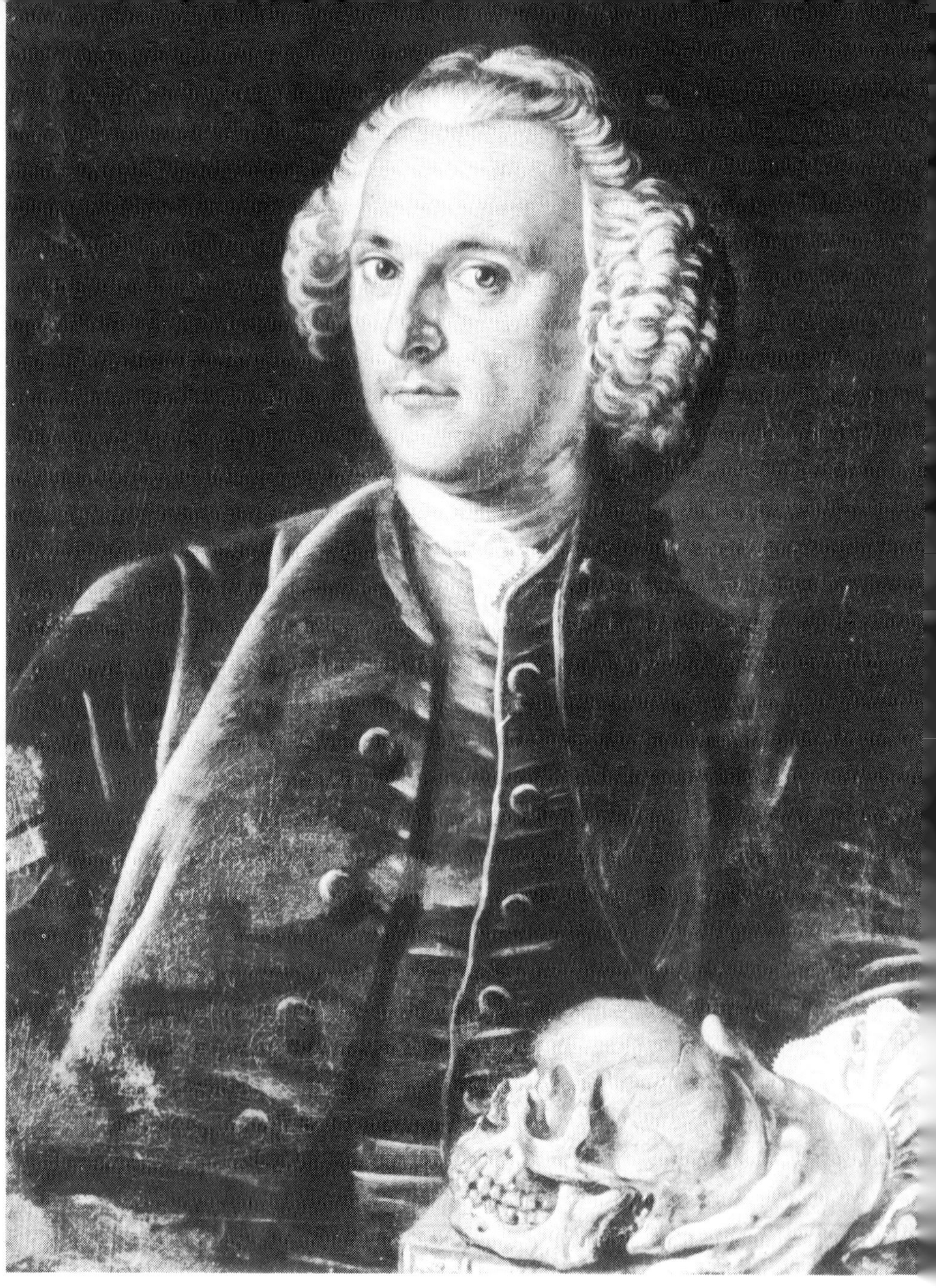

Plate 1 Jan Van Rymsdyk's portrait of William Barrett, painted in 1764. (City of Bristol Museum and Art Gallery).

went to Belle Isle and Portugal on active service in 1761. Jenty stayed there when the expedition returned to England in 1763, but John Hunter was now back in London, and William Hunter was also in need of an artist. Rymsdyk must have swallowed his pride, for in 1764 he made at least nine drawings for the *Gravid uterus,* followed by others in successive years up to 1772. He probably had other work on hand, and in 1767 he made a mezzotint engraving of Frederick Henry and Emilia Van Solms, Prince and Princess of Orange, from a painting by Jordaens at Devonshire House.

During this period Rymsdyk must have saved his money, and instead of the penury to which he had been reduced in Bristol, we find him embarking upon an ambitious work, to be financed by himself. In July, 1772, he applied to the British Museum for permission to draw birds and other exhibits, with the idea of publishing *Museum Britannicum.* In this venture he was to be assisted by his son Andrew, who made drawings for some of the illustrations (see Chapter 7). Jan Van Rymsdyk was responsible for the majority of these, and for the text, but he did not do the engraving, although he was capable of this, as evidenced by the fact that he engraved one of the plates in Hunter's *Gravid uterus.* In September 1775, he was advertising for "Engravers who understand to imitate chalk drawings", but *Museum Britannicum* was not finally published until 1778 (see Chapter 6).

Although Jan Van Rymsdyk had asserted in this book that he no longer intended to draw medical subjects, he also complained about the high cost of the venture, and by 1783 he was obviously experiencing the need for earning money. His son had gone to Bath as a miniature-portrait painter, but died in 1786, and the *Museum Britannicum* was probably not as remunerative as anticipated. William Hunter had died in 1783, and John Hunter installed an artist on his premises in 1775. Probably neither would have employed Rymsdyk following the publication of his book, but he found a new patron in Thomas Denman (1733–1815), (see Chapter 8). Several drawings were executed for Denman between 1783 and 1788, the last being published on 23 February 1789. A second edition of *Museum Britannicum,* edited by Peter Boyle, was published in 1791, and Jan Van Rymsdyk was certainly dead by then; he most probably died in 1788 or 1789. He disappeared as mysteriously as he had arrived in London in 1750, for no record of his passing has been traced. His work, as recorded in the following chapters, remains as his monument, and no medical artist could anticipate greater appreciation than the fact that his work is still admired two hundred years after it was executed.

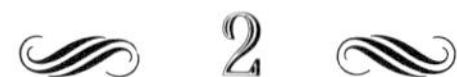

2

RYMSDYK'S DRAWINGS FOR WILLIAM SMELLIE (1697–1763)

"Then came Smellie's 'Tables' in 1754 and Hunter's 'Gravid uterus' in 1774 and a revolution in obstetrical book production had occurred which certainly affected other branches of surgery and medicine. This magnificent elephant folio and the tables of William Smellie have never been equalled; they are the masterpieces of their time and were harbingers of a new era in medical illustration."

Alistair L. Gunn (1967-68).

William Smellie (1697–1763), described by his biographer R. W. Johnstone (1952) as "the master of British midwifery", was the outstanding obstetrician of the eighteenth century, and his influence has persisted to the present day. He was born in 1697, probably in Lanark, the only child of Archibald and Sara Smellie. Educated at the local grammar school, he acquired a working knowledge of Latin and probably French. He entered the medical profession by apprenticeship to Dr. John Gordon of Glasgow, and settled as a medical practitioner in his native town, initially without any other medical qualification. Smellie practised in Lanark from 1720 to 1739, and in 1724 he married Eupham Borland, but they had no children. His father died in 1735, presumably leaving his estate to William, and the following year he purchased a house in Bloomgate, and two pieces of land outside the town. About 1733 William Smellie became a member of the Faculty of Physicians and Surgeons of Glasgow, and twelve years later was granted an M.D. by the University of Glasgow.

In 1739 William Smellie went to London, apparently to acquire further knowledge regarding the use of obstetrical forceps, but he found little information available there, and proceeded to Paris. He attended the lectures of Gregoire, but was again disappointed in his quest, although he picked up the idea of using the "phantom" for teaching purposes. Returning to London, Smellie settled in a modest house in Pall Mall as an apothecary and practitioner of midwifery, but moved first to Gerrard Street and then Wardour Street. He attended lectures on natural philosophy by Desaguliers, and on normal and morbid anatomy by Frank Nicholls (1699–1778). In his first year he received William Hunter into his house for several months, and probably both derived professional benefit from the experience. They were fellow Scots, but later their paths diverged, Smellie to work among the poorer classes, while William Hunter built up a practice in higher circles, including royalty.

Smellie began to teach midwifery in 1741, and the *London Evening Post* for 1 June 1742 advertised his lectures on the subject for both women and men, but at different times. Smellie and his students attended poor women in their own homes, and he made students pay six shillings each into a fund for the support of needy patients. Although there was great antagonism towards men-midwives, Smellie not only practised the art but openly instructed both men and women. He was attacked in pamphlets by several writers, including Mrs. Nihell, Philip Thickness, John Burton, and William Douglas, but he deigned to reply only to Douglas. It has been estimated by S. J. Cameron (1957) that during ten years in London, Smellie gave 280 courses in midwifery, each lasting a fortnight, to over nine hundred pupils, and that during that period over eleven hundred poor women were delivered.

William Smellie contributed to the improvement of obstetric forceps by shortening and lightening the whole instrument, by inventing the "lock", by applying the pelvic curve, and by formulating rules for their use. At one time he employed wooden forceps, and then leather wrapping around the blades, but he did suggest that this should be renewed after each case. He was never on the staff of a lying-in hospital, and never attended a woman of rank, confining his attention to the poor in their homes.

In 1759 Smellie arranged for his teaching to be continued by Dr. John Harvie, a former pupil, and returned to Lanark for the last three years of his life, which he spent gathering together records of preternatural labour for the third volume of his *Treatise on the theory and practice of midwifery.* Having completed this, he sent it to his friend Tobias Smollett (1721–1771), who provided the literary polish to the work, but Smellie did not live to see it published. He died on 5 March 1763 and was buried in his parents' grave in St. Kentigern at Lanark. He and his wife made a joint Will in 1759, to become operative after the death of both. The estate was mainly left to Mrs. Smellie's niece Anne, who had married John Harvie, but Smellie's books and certain other effects, together with two hundred pounds, were left to the School at Lanark. After many years of neglect, the books were restored by Miles Phillips

(1875–1965) and are now in the custody of the County Librarian in the Lindsay Institute in Lanark. A recent survey of the history of Smellie's Library is provided by Antonia J. Bunch (1975, pp. 65–72), which supplements an earlier study by H. P. Tait and A. T. Wallace (1952).

In his joint Will, which is reproduced in the definitive biography by John Glaister (1894, pp. 323–328), Smellie also left to the School at Lanark some furniture, musical instruments, music books and three pictures which hung in his study: "My father's, mother's and my own, drawn by myself in 1719". Some mystery surrounds these pictures, which were thought to have "disappeared" from the Grammar School. From the wording of the Will one might infer that Smellie painted all three portraits, but those of his parents were possibly painted by John Smellie. It is thought that the self-portrait never went to the School, and in 1828 the Royal College of Surgeons of Edinburgh received as a gift from Mr. John Harvie, Writer to the Signet, a portrait of the late Dr. Smellie. This was later pronounced to be the "original picture painted by Smellie himself and not a copy" (Glaister (1894), pp. 336), which suggests that the father of the donor had not carried out the stipulation in Smellie's Will, of which he was executor. In 1932 a copy of this portrait was made by David Alison for Miles Phillips and R. W. Johnstone, and this was presented to the Royal College of Obstetricians and Gynaecologists, London. In fact, it appears probable that two copies were made, as Miles Phillips, writing in 1954 stated that one was hanging in his study over his head, and had been there since October 1932. This was intended to be placed later with Smellie's library in the Lindsay Institute, but its present location has not been discovered.

In 1753 Jan Van Rymsdyk painted or drew a portrait of William Smellie, but the original of this has not been found. It was engraved by Charles Grignion, and even the engraving is very rare, copies having been traced only in the Royal College of Physicians of London and the University of Edinburgh (Plate 2).

The writings of William Smellie extended the range of his teaching, and their popularity ensured that they were reprinted several times. They were also made available in French, Dutch and German translations. The first volume was published as *A treatise on the theory and practice of midwifery,* London, dated 1752, but actually issued in 1751 (see McClintock's edition, p. 22), and the second volume followed in 1754, with the sub-title *A collection of cases and observations in midwifery, to illustrate his former treatise.* Volume three was published the year after Smellie's death, with the sub-title *A collection of preternatural cases and observations in midwifery compleating the design of illustrating the first volume on that subject*, 1764. These were all prepared for the press by his friend Tobias Smollett. In 1876 the New Sydenham Society published the three-volume edition, edited by Alfred H. McClintock

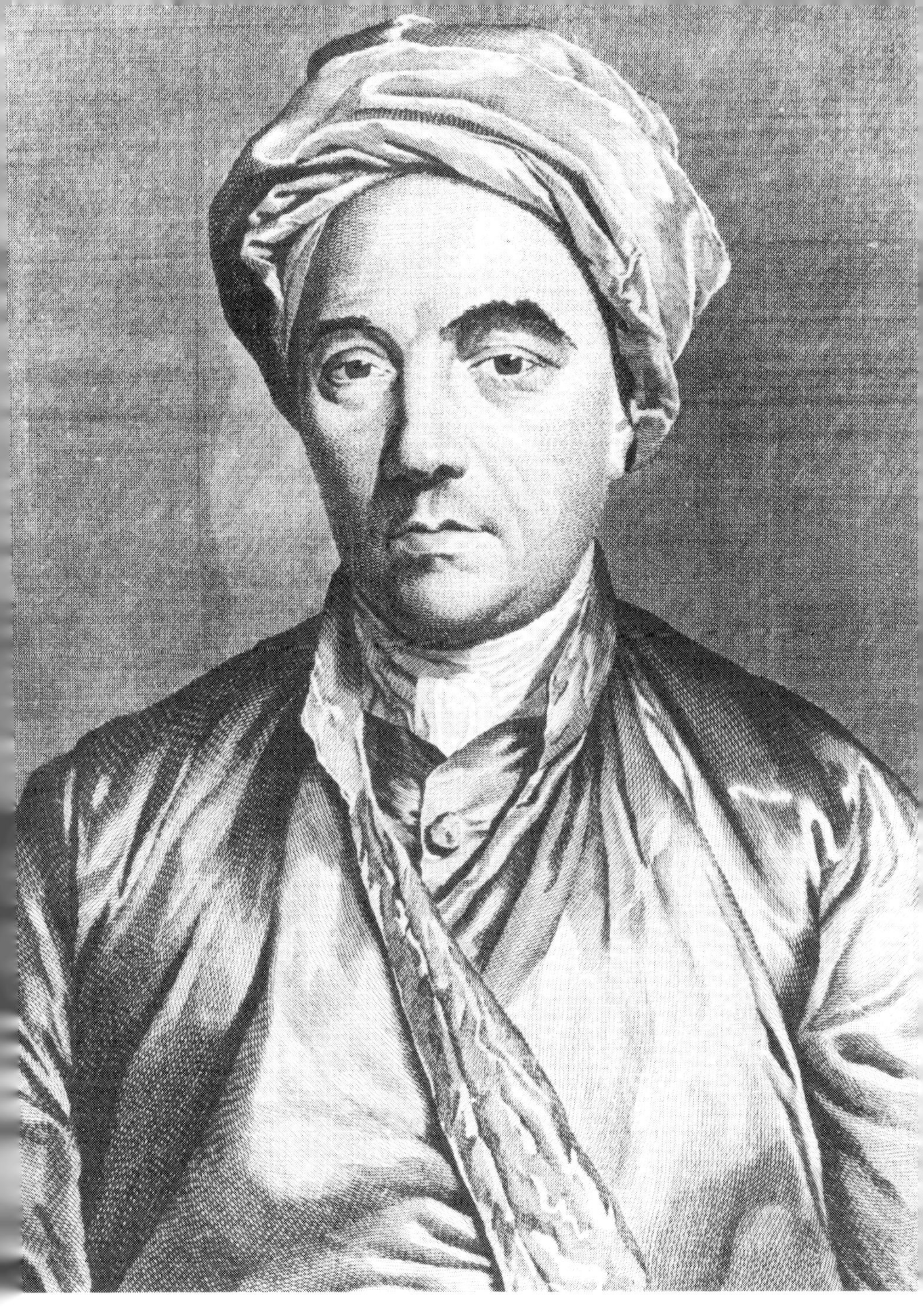

Plate 2 Engraving by Charles Grignion of Jan Van Rymsdyk's portrait of William Smellie, painted or drawn in 1753. (Royal College of Physicians of London).

(1822–1881) from the Edinburgh, 1788 edition, with practical, historical and critical annotations.

In the preface to the first volume of his *Treatise* Smellie stated:

> "It was my intention to insert in this Compendium, plates of the most useful instruments appertaining to the art of Midwifery; but as large drawings could not be properly bound in a book of so small a size, I have resolved to publish them in folio, with that set of prints which I am now preparing, according to the proposals specified in the advertisement at the end of this volume." (p. vi).

The advertisement occupies nine pages, and commences:

> "Doctor *Smellie* having, with great care and expence, employed Mr. *Riemsdyk* to draw anatomical figures, as large as the human subjects themselves, for the use of those who attend his lectures, and in order to illustrate his theory and practice of midwifery; and being desirous to render his drawings of more extensive and general use, by causing them to be engraved by able artists, a design which cannot be put in execution without a considerable expence; he proposes to publish the whole set by subscription, in the following manner:
>
> I.
>
> The work will consist of twenty-six plates, of about 18 inches by 12.
>
> II.
>
> A full and distinct explanation of each plate will be printed on a large sheet, of the same size with the figures, that they may be bound up together. For the use of foreigners, there will also be an explanation printed in *Latin,* and a list of the subscribers shall be published, if desired.
>
> III.
>
> The price to subscribers will be two guineas, one to be paid at the time of subscribing, and the other at the delivery of the prints, with their explanation.
>
> IV.
>
> The drawings will be put into the hands of the best engravers, as soon as a number of subscriptions are received sufficient to defray the expence of the work, which will be executed with as great dispatch as shall be consistent with the nature and accuracy of the performance."

This is followed by descriptions of the proposed twenty-six plates, and concludes:

> "Subscriptions are taken in by D. Wilson, the publisher, at *Plato's* head, near *Round-Court,* in the *Strand,* where two of the drawings are to be seen, as specimens of the work; as also by the booksellers of *Britain* and *Ireland, France* and *Holland* where proposals, with lists of the prints, are to be had."

It is obvious from this that Smellie's atlas had been planned at the same time as his Treatise, and that some of the illustrations had already been drawn by Rymsdyk and engraved. However, the arrangement of the plates was changed, and the number of plates was increased to thirty-nine, some later editions containing forty or forty-one. Smellie's *A sett (sic) of anatomical tables with explanations and an abridgement of the practice of midwifery, with a view to illustrate a Treatise on the subject,* London, was published in 1754. Incidentally, the spelling "sett" in the title is not an example of old English, but was a misprint, as noted in the errata at the end of the book. In his preface Smellie explained that he was attempting to explain what he had taught and written, and continues:

> ". . . the greatest part of the figures were taken from Subjects prepared on purpose to show everything that might conduce to the improvement of the young Practitioner, avoiding, however, the extreme Minutiae. . . the situation of parts and their respective dimensions being more particularly attended to than a minute anatomical investigation of their structure. . .
>
> My first plan for these Tables confined them to the number of twenty-two, which Mr. Rymsdyke had finished above two years ago; but I saw that. . . an addition to that number was necessary. In eleven of these Dr. Camper. . . greatly assisted me, viz. Table XII, XVI, XVII, XVIII, XIX, XXIV, XXVI, XXVII, XXVIII, XXXIV, and XXXVI. The rest were drawn by Mr. Rymsdyke; except the thirty-seventh and thirty-ninth, which were done by another hand. The Whole of the Drawings were faithfully engraved (by Mr. Grignion); in which, however, delicacy and elegance have not been so much consulted as to have them done in a strong and distinct manner; with this view chiefly, that from the cheapness of the work it may be rendered of more general use."

It has been assumed that "by another hand" obscures the identity of Smellie himself, and that being no mean artist, he was probably the originator of Tables XXXVII and XXXIX. However, as noted below, the original drawings for Camper's eleven plates, and twenty-five by Rymsdyk, still exist, which leaves Table XXXVIII unaccounted for. As this is one of the series of drawings of instruments, featuring a fillet and pessaries, and catheters, it appears probable that the same artist was responsible for these figures, and it is significant that the original drawings for Table XXXVIII is not preserved with the drawings by either Rymsdyk or Camper.

Pieter (Petrus) Camper (1722–1789) visited England three times, the first in 1748 when he came to study art and midwifery. In January 1749 he enrolled for Smellie's course in midwifery, and in 1752, by now Professor of Medicine at Franeker, he visited Smellie and was shown Rymsdyk's drawings. It was on this occasion that Camper "greatly assisted" Smellie. He dissected, and made drawings, most of the originals of which are signed "Camper" and dated 1752. These are now housed in the Library of the Royal College of Physicians of Edinburgh, to which they were presented, bound in a folio, by Dr. G. M. Burt. The University of Leyden has seven similar drawings, all signed by Camper, but it has been determined that those at Edinburgh are the originals for Smellie's *Tables,* and that Camper probably made the other copies for his own use (see Johnstone, 1952, pp. 88–89). Camper was appointed Professor of Anatomy and Surgery at Amsterdam in 1775, and among other works published a book on the connection between the science of anatomy and the arts of drawing, painting and statuary. Camper's last visit to England was made in 1785, and he left an interesting diary recording his activities during the three visits (Camper, 1939). This mentions places visited by Camper, gives the names of the distinguished people he met, but gives no indication that he had any direct contact with his fellow countryman, Jan Van Rymsdyk, although he did see the drawings executed by Rymsdyk for both Smellie and William Hunter. Possibly there was a marked distinction between the social classes, and Rymsdyk was regarded as a craftsman or tradesman, not to be mixed with socially. To Camper he may also have appeared as a refugee; to William Hunter, just another employé.

Camper gives details of many midwifery cases he visited with Smellie, and also provides annotations to his course of lectures, which he first attended during his visit when he recorded that on 5 January 1749 "I subscribed on Dr. Smellie's course of midwifery for three guineas". During his second visit in 1752 he notes for July:

> "On Friday morning the 14th I hired two rooms in Meards Buildings near Dr. Smellie, who was the first person I saw, as also his figures drawn by Rymsdijk, but not all from real life. The children were placed in pelves of women, the children themselves looked natural, but the other parts were copied from other preparations. What I thought very good was the way the bones were drawn over the children with white dots. The drawings were done in vermilion on a yellow background." (p. 121)
>
> "On Tuesday I drew for Smellie, and checked precisely the position

of the heads that are wedged. Wednesday at Smellie's, dined at Hunter's and saw his figures of uterus gravidus, which are very beautiful, drawn bij (sic) Rymsdijk. He had prepared it and afterwards moulded it in plaster, which I think a very good idea, which I shall apply in future." (p. 123).

"Friday 21st I drew for Smellie and with the forceps delivered from a corpse a head in a transversal position wedged with the ear against the os pubis." (p. 125) (August 31st)". . . Dr. Smellie was with me that evening we saw the copperplate, engraved by Grinson (*sic* Grignion) which we both much admired. He told me he was going to continue with those relating to the forceps." (p. 165).

There are twelve original drawings by Camper at Edinburgh, but only eleven were engraved for Smellie's *Atlas,* the one omitted being similar to Table XII, but with the head of the fetus lower in the pelvis. Most of the drawings are mainly diagrammatic, and the engravings by Grignion were embellished with more detail. Although Camper had seen Rymsdyk's drawings, he certainly made no attempt to equal their artistic merit, and it is possible that Smellie instructed him to include only such detail as was necessary to his immediate purpose. This was mainly to indicate the position of the fetus in the uterus, and the application of the forceps to the head. It would appear that Camper's drawings for Smellie were all made in 1752, probably after Rymsdyk had completed his series, and that the latter was engaged on other work. Also, Smellie was anxious to have his *Atlas* published as soon as possible to accompany his *Treatise.* We have found no evidence to support suggestions that Camper made some drawings for Smellie in 1749, and continued the series in 1752, nor that he sent Rymsdyk to Smellie from Holland as a replacement for himself as an artist.

The first eleven of the plates drawn by Rymsdyk show the anatomy of the pelvis; a distorted pelvis; the external genitalia; the internal generative organs; the pregnant uterus opened at the second/third and fourth/fifth months; a twin pregnancy; and the partially dissected uterus at term (Plate 3). Tables thirteen and fourteen depict progressively later stages in natural labour, and the next plate illustrates the application of forceps to the head. Table fifteen shows the perineum and external parts stretched by the head of the fetus, and in Table twenty the forehead of the fetus is turned towards the pubes. Table twenty-one is similar to the previous one, but with the forceps in position, (Plate 4), and Table twenty-two shows the forehead of the fetus presenting a lateral view of the face of the child presenting, and forced down into the lower part of the pelvis. A similar position is shown in Table twenty-five, but with the chin to the

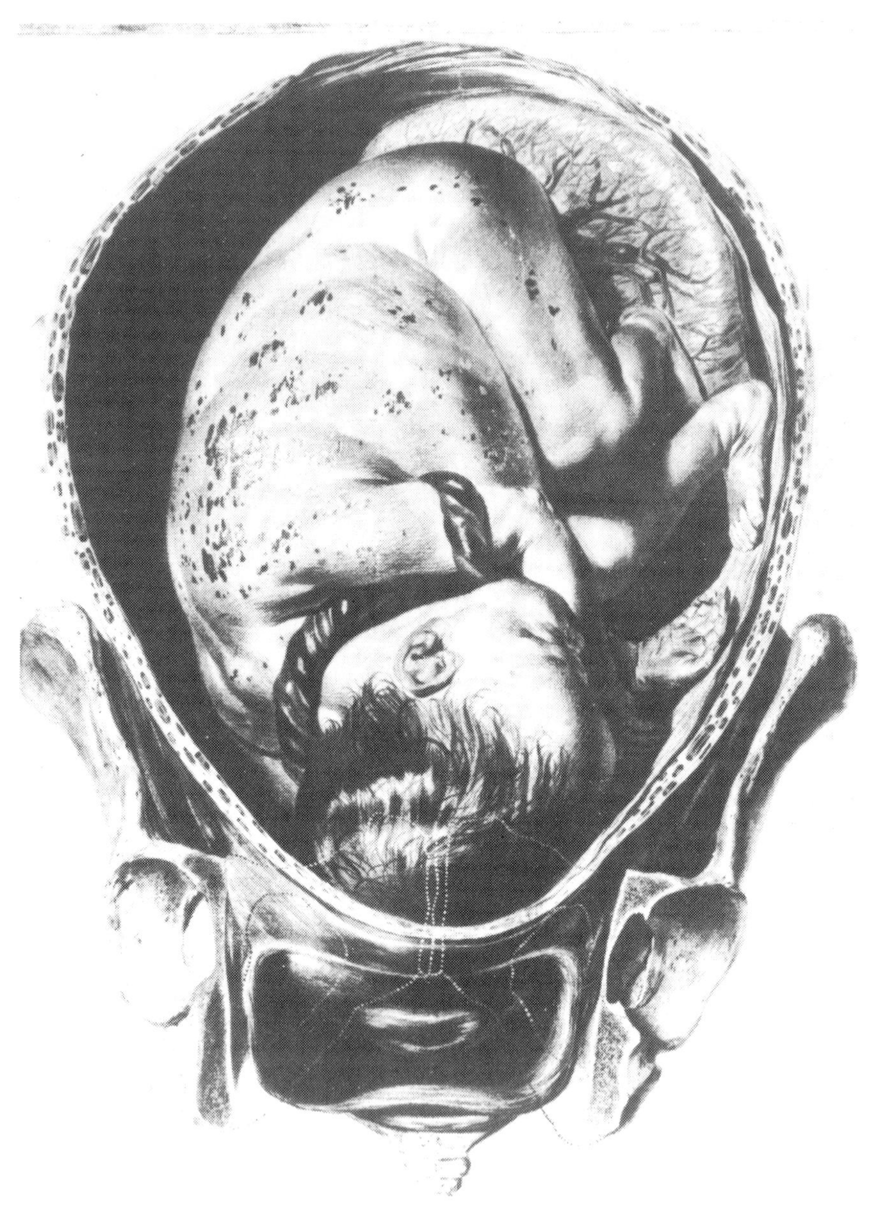

Plate 3 Rymsdyk's original drawing of the gravid uterus in the eighth or ninth month of pregnancy. Engraved as Table 9 in Smellie's *Sett of anatomical tables,* 1754. (Hunterian Collection, Glasgow).

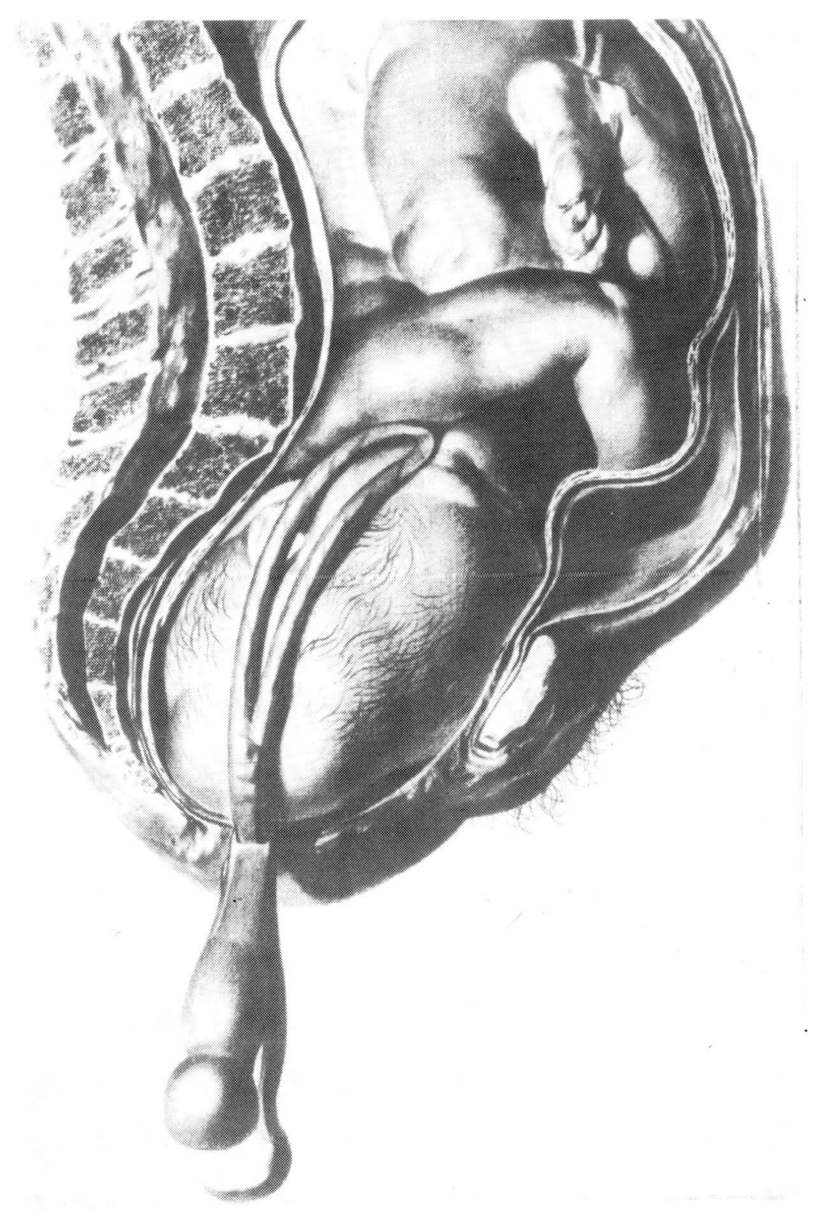

Plate 4 Rymsdyk's original drawing of Smellie's forceps in position around head of fetus. Engraved as Table 21 in Smellie's *Sett of anatomical tables,* 1754. (Hunterian Collection, Glasgow).

os sacrum, and the bregma to the pubes. A breech presentation is featured in Table twenty-nine, with the cord knotted around the neck, arm and body. Table thirty also shows a breech presentation, but with the fore-part of the child to the fore-part of the uterus. In Table thirty-one the fetus is compressed into circular form, with one foot and hand descended into the vagina. Table thirty-two is similar, but the forearm is outside the os externum, and the shoulder is forced into the os uteri. This position of the fetus is repeated in Table thirty-three, but with the umbilical region presenting at the os internum, the cord appearing at the os externum. Table thirty-five is a lateral view of the pelvis, showing the method of assisting delivery of the head with long curved forceps in praeternatural cases. Several of the original drawings have the pelvis dotted in, this feature being omitted in the engravings.

Although Smellie's *Atlas* bears the date 1754, the *General Evening Post* dated 22 July 1755 carries the following advertisement:

> "*This Day were published,* (Price £2.5s. in sheets) THIRTY-SIX TABLES OF ANATOMICAL FIGURES, as large as the Human Subjects, and Three of INSTRUMENTS, to illustrate Dr. SMELLIE's Treatise and Cases in Midwifery, engraved by Mr. Grignion, from the Drawings of Mr. Riemsdyk and others, with an explanation to each Figure on fine large Imperial Paper. N.B. The Subscribers are desired to send their Receipts and second Payments
> Street, Soho; or to D. Wilson and T. Durham, at Plato's Head in the Strand; where the Books are delivered; and where may be had Dr. Smellie's Midwifery, in 2 vols. Price 12s. bound.
>
> ☞ The Doctor begins a new Course of Lectures on Monday the 4th of August".

Dr. John Harvie succeeded William Smellie as teacher of midwifery in Wardour Street, and after Harvie's death his teaching material was sold at an auction in 1770. Rymsdyk's twenty-five original drawings were sold as one lot, which was purchased by William Hunter, and at his death they were left with his other magnificent collections to the University of Glasgow. The drawings are in "sanguine" coloured chalk, (also described as red, sepia, etc.) and are finished in a masterly manner, although they are not as detailed as those executed for William Hunter. Smellie's aim was to produce something very akin to the diagrammatic illustrations in later textbooks, while Hunter's idea was to have drawings of strict accuracy and artistic excellence never previously achieved.

When William Smellie finally left London, William Hunter, William Osborn and Thomas Denman became his successors, and none of these was enthusiastic about the use of forceps. Smellie's teaching was still appreciated in

Scotland and on the Continent, but in England it suffered a temporary eclipse. His contributions are the better appreciated by a study of John Glaister's *Dr. William Smellie and his contemporaries. A contribution to the history of midwifery in the eigteenth century,* Glasgow, 1894. This is a very thorough biography, and includes chapters on "Conditions of midwifery in London at this period"; "His first critic – William Douglas"; "Progress of midwifery teaching in London"; "Smellie's friends"; "Literature of midwifery from 1660–1760"; "Forceps before and during Smellie's time"; "Burton on Smellie"; "Scottish graduates in London"; "Smellie and the opponents of man-midwifery"; "Other critics of Smellie"; with an appendix including a Bibliography of his works. It contains twenty-nine illustrations and a photogravure portrait of Smellie from the original at the Royal College of Surgeons, Edinburgh. A shorter modern biography was written by R. W. Johnstone (1879–1969) and published as *William Smellie: the master of British midwifery,* Edinburgh, London, 1952. This shorter study brings the subject more up to date, and being more concise, is more readily readable as an introduction to the life and work of this great pioneer. Although out of print, it is still more readily available than that by Glaister, of which only five hundred copies were printed.

Smellie's writings were reprinted and translated on many occasions, and the plates from his atlas were copied without acknowledgement even more frequently. In 1971 the University of Auckland issued a beautifully produced reprint of the *Anatomical tables,* making it more generally available than the original edition, copies of which command a high price.

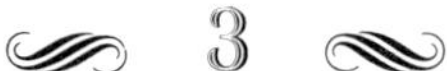

RYMSDYK'S DRAWINGS FOR WILLIAM HUNTER (1718–1783)

> *"These thirty-four copperplates represent the gravid uterus and its contents in life-size, anatomically exact, and artistically perfect."*
>
> Ludwig Choulant.

Although Rymsdyk's drawings for Smellie were the first to be published in book form, he probably began his series for William Hunter before embarking on those for Smellie. Hunter's *Gravid uterus* was not printed until 1774, but Rymsdyk started on the initial drawings in 1750, when he first appeared in London. In addition to the illustrations for that book, he made many other drawings for William Hunter, all of which are preserved in the Hunterian Collection at Glasgow University. This contains a wealth of material relating to William Hunter, together with his extensive collection of books, manuscripts, coins, pictures and specimens, but it has not been as extensively exploited as that of his brother John Hunter at the Royal College of Surgeons in London. Both men have been the subjects of numerous lectures and writings, but William has not been the subject of a definitive biography. Richard Hingston Fox (1901) and George Charles Peachey (1924) are very useful sources of information, but Sir Charles Illingworth's *The story of William Hunter,* 1967, written in the form of an autobiography, is a mixture of fact and fiction, making it an unreliable source for the serious historian. Probably the best biogaphy of William Hunter is contained in the Introduction (pp. xxi–lxxvii) to John H. Teacher's *Catalogue of the anatomical and pathological preparations of Dr. William Hunter in the Hunterian Museum, University of Glasgow,* two volumes, 1900, which was reproduced (pp. xxi–lxxvii) in Alice J. Marshall's *Catalogue,* 1970. This is in one volume, and is confined to the anatomical preparations. Alistair Gunn (1967–8) also published a very interesting Hunterian Oration, with useful information on both John and William Hunter.

The main events of William Hunter's life, with emphasis on those appertaining to his obstetrical career, are here outlined in an attempt to indicate the influence of others on his particular interest in the subject. They also suggest the gradual development of his knowledge of the growth of the fetus, and explain why his atlas devoted to the gravid uterus, planned at least as early as 1750, was not finally published until 1774.

William Hunter was born at Long Calderwood near East Kilbride on 23 May 1718 and became a student in the Faculty of Arts at Glasgow University. His father had intended him to enter the Church, but in 1737 he went to live with William Cullen (1710–1790) at Hamilton and remained his apprentice for three years. Cullen greatly influenced Hunter's career, and they remained great friends throughout life. Some of the correspondence between them is printed in the biography of Cullen by John Thomson (1859). In 1740 Hunter attended the anatomical lectures of Alexander Monro (1697–1767) in Edinburgh, then the following year travelled by sea to London, with letters of introduction to William Smellie, James Douglas and several other Scotsmen. After living with Smellie for a few weeks, Hunter went to reside with Douglas as assistant, and as tutor to his son.

Although his stay with William Smellie was brief, Hunter probably derived great benefit from the association, being introduced to midwifery among the poorer classes. Smellie was content to confine his practice to these, and was probably not of the same social standing as William Hunter. However, they respected each other, and Hunter attended several of Smellie's cases.

James Douglas (1675–1742) was very versatile: a physician, obstetrician, anatomist, natural historian, grammarian and student of Horace. His influence on William Hunter extended beyond his life, as Hunter inherited his manuscripts and drawings. Hunter lived in the Douglas household as tutor to William George Douglas, who later gave up medicine, and died in 1755 aged about thirty. Apparently Hunter was attracted to Martha Jane Douglas, but she died in 1744 aged twenty-eight. William Hunter's younger brother James also joined the household in 1742, but his health failed, and he returned to Long Calderwood, to die on 11 April 1745. Later, John Hunter also lived briefly in the Douglas household, but then moved with William Hunter to the Great Piazza in Covent Garden.

In addition to his published work, James Douglas left many unfinished manuscripts and drawings, including copper-plates and proofs of a book on osteology. When he died on 1 April 1742, James Douglas had accomplished much, but had many other projects in hand, and left material which came into William Hunter's possession, and is now in the Hunterian Collection at Glasgow. K. Bryn Thomas (1964) has studied the relationship between

Douglas and Hunter in a book which also contains both "An annotated catalogue of the manuscripts and drawings of James Douglas and others", and a list of his publications. This book was later supplemented by a significant paper by Helen Brock (1974), which confirms that James Douglas is worthy of more extensive study, and that the value of his work has not achieved full recognition. It does appear obvious, however, that his studies of many subjects affected the future interests of the two Hunters, both of whom, for example, later pursued his keen interest in the development of the chick embryo. His interest in the gravid uterus also probably initiated William Hunter's later work on the subject.

As tutor to William Douglas, Hunter had accompanied him to Paris and to Holland, and it is apparent that Hunter derived more from these excursions than did his pupil. James Douglas also encouraged Hunter to study surgery at St. George's Hospital under James Wilkie, and anatomy under Frank Nicholls. William Hunter continued to live in the Douglas household after the death of his patron, and he determined to become a teacher of anatomy. He opened a school first located in Covent Garden, then in Jermyn Street, and finally, in 1771, in a specially erected building later known as the Great Windmill Street School of Anatomy.

William Hunter had been admitted a member of the Corporation of Surgeons in 1747, and a year later was a "surgeon accoucheur" to Middlesex Hospital. In 1749 he held a similar post at the British Lying-in Hospital, but having obtained the Glasgow M.D. in 1750, and been disfranchised from the Corporation of Surgeons in July 1756, he was admitted a licentiate of the College of Physicians in September of that year. He then gave up any connection with gynaecological surgery; his brief career in this connection with the lying-in hospitals is recorded by George C. Peachey (1930). Hunter now concentrated on building up his school of anatomy and extending his midwifery practice, the latter being greatly advanced when in 1762 he attended Queen Charlotte in her first confinement; two years later he was appointed her Physician Extraordinary. A diary written by William Hunter during his attendance at the first three accouchements of Queen Charlotte has been edited with notes by J. Nigel Stark (1908) from which it is obvious that his services were confined to attention after the actual birth, Mrs. Draper being the midwife who conducted the proceedings. Hunter's original account is preserved in the Hunterian Museum, Glasgow.

The Royal Academy of Arts was founded on 10 December 1768, and the Instrument of Foundation signed by George III decreed that "there shall be a Professor of Anatomy, who shall read annually six public lectures in the Schools, adapted to the Arts of Design; his salary shall be thirty pounds a year;

and he shall continue in office during the King's pleasure." A week later William Hunter was appointed to the Chair of Anatomy, and on 27 December 1769 a resolution of Council decided "that Dr. Wm. Hunter (as Anatomy Professor) have free access to all General Assembly's." From 1769 to 1772 Hunter kept rough notes and drafts on envelopes, letters etc. of his lectures at the Academy, which have been edited by Martin Kemp (1975).

William Hunter's first published paper was read to the Royal Society on 2 June 1743, and was printed in its *Philosophical Transactions* (volume 42, 1742/3 (1744), pp. 514–521) and nothing further was published under his name until 1757. In 1754 he became a member of the Society of Physicians, forerunner of the London Medical Society, and in 1757 appeared the first of the six published volumes of its transactions, under the title *Medical Observations and Inquiries,* and Hunter's first of a sequence of papers was printed therein. Others appeared in the *Philosophical Transactions*, and a bibliography of all William Hunter's papers and books was published by W. R. LeFanu (1958), supplemented by A. L. Goodall (1958). These record the various editions, reprints and translations.

The study of embryology and the gravid uterus was not undertaken by the very early anatomists, and A. H. F. Barbour (1888) has briefly outlined the history of the subject. Hippocrates (*c.* 450–*c.* 370 B.C.) dissected animals only, and the idea prevailed that the human uterus consisted of two cavities. Aristotle (*c.* 384–322 B.C.) held the same views, and stated that males developed in the right half of the uterus, and females in the left. Soranus of Ephesus (98–138 A.D.) provided a good account of the organs of generation in his *Gynaecia,* which survives in the original Greek, and of which there are Latin, French, German and English translations. His ideas were revived by later writers for several centuries. Galen (130–200 A.D.) attempted to describe organs he had never observed, but apparently he had never opened a female pelvis. Muscio, or Moschion, who is believed to have flourished about 500 A.D., followed the teaching of Soranus, and wrote a catechism with 152 questions and answers which was first published in 1566 in Caspar Wolff's *Gynaeciorum,* and contains what was thought to be the earliest drawing of the human uterus. Mondino de' Luzzi, or Mundinus (*c.* 1276–1326) taught anatomy in Bologna, and dissected several female bodies, but apparently did not examine the uterus, which he described as containing seven cavities. His *Anothomia* was written for his students in 1316 and first published in 1487, but is very defective on female pelvic anatomy.

Leonardo da Vinci (1452–1519) established an intimate relationship between art and anatomy, and it is most unfortunate that the brilliance of his anatomical and embryological drawings could not be appreciated until centuries after his death. William Hunter saw the drawings in the collection of George III at Windsor in 1773 (Martin Kemp, 1976), and intended to publish them, but died before this was accomplished.

Giacomo Berengario da Carpi (*c.* 1460–1530) dissected at least a hundred bodies, and his *Isagogae breves,* (*etc.*), Bologna, 1522, went into numerous editions and translations. This book introduced art to anatomical illustration, and the subjects are represented as if alive. A female stands in front of a veil, the abdomen laid open, showing the uterus and cervix divided coronally. She holds in her right hand the front half of these, and the book also contains a plate of the uterus. Andreas Vesalius (1514–1564) is rightly regarded as the founder of scientific anatomy, and his *De humani corporis fabrica libri septem,* Basle, 1543, with a second edition in 1555, is a masterpiece in the history of anatomy and anatomical illustration. Several figures illustrate the uterus, and Figure 30 represents the pregnant uterus when laid open. Bartholomew Eustachius (1520–1574) made numerous valuable contributions to anatomical knowledge, and at his death left thirty-eight copper-plates for an unpublished book which he had completed in 1552. These were published by Giovanni Lancisi (1654–1720) as *Tabulae anatomicae,* Rome, 1714, which includes two plates of the uterus, one featuring the fetus with chorion and amnion.

The next contributions to the anatomy of the female organs of generation were made by Gabriele Fallopius (1523–1562) in his *Observationes anatomicae,* Venice, 1561, in which he describes the clitoris and hymen, the uterus, round ligaments, ovaries, the "Fallopian" tubes, and the anatomy of the pregnant uterus, describing the placenta. Regnier de Graaf (1641–1673) first described the "Graafian follicles" in *De mulierum organis generatione inservientibus tractatus novus,* Leyden, 1672. Albrecht von Haller (1708–1777) studied under Boerhaave, and made important contributions to anatomy, botany, medicine and physiology. In 1727 he came to England and met James Douglas and other distinguished medical men. Haller had also dissected in Paris with Bernhard Siegfried Albinus (1697–1770), the author of *Icones ossium foetus humani,* Leyden, 1737, and of *Tabulae septem uteri mulieris gravidae cum jam parturiret mortuae,* Leyden, 1747, which contains seven plates of the gravid uterus. The anatomical atlases of Albinus are noted for the beauty of the figures drawn and engraved by Jan Wandelaer (1690–1759), which were all measured and brought down to scale. Abraham Vater (1684–1751) was the author of *Dissertatio anatomico-pathologica qua uterus gravidus physiologice et pathologice consideratur exposita simul eius structura et orificiorum menses at lochia fundentium fabrica sistitur,* Wittenberg, 1725, which contains a drawing of the pregnant uterus at six months. The *Icones uteri humani observationibus illustratae,* Göttingen, 1757, has seven plates of the gravid uterus, and was written by Johann Georg Roederer (1727–1763).

These indicate the slow development of investigations into female anatomy, which gained impetus with the spread of dissection and the teaching of increasing numbers of medical students. These required access to textbooks, particularly those containing illustrations, and the atlases in particular were very popular. The older books were not readily available, and this prompted teachers to provide their own textbooks, and particularly to make the texts available in English as well as other languages, especially in Latin, then the international language for medicine.

Childbirth and the attendant difficulties received increasing attention with the development of scientific knowledge, and with an appreciation of the need for the replacement of the ignorant midwife by skilled professionals. This implied that they should have a knowledge of female internal anatomy, of embryological development, of the mechanics of childbirth, and of the problems associated with abnormal deliveries and the postpartem period. The acquisition of this knowledge was a slow process, hampered by religious objections, by reluctance to permit men to act as midwives, and by the attitude of the medical profession towards fellow-members of the profession who wanted to specialise in obstetrics and gynaecology. These prejudices still persist to some extent, and the man-midwife has struggled for over three hundred years for acceptance as a specialist by profession.

William Smellie was probably the first to teach midwifery to both men and women, (in separate classes of course), and it is of interest to note that James Douglas, William Hunter and C. N. Jenty all planned books on the gravid uterus within the space of a few years. Smellie's book (see Chapter 2) was the first to be printed, but that by William Hunter required a gestation period of twenty-four years.

The bicentenary of the publication of William Hunter's *The anatomy of the human gravid uterus* was noted by the publication of articles by Robert Ollerenshaw (1974) and by Thornton and Patricia C. Want (1974), both of which contain information on those associated with the production of the book, which has held its place as a masterpiece of technical skill for over two hundred years (Plate 5). Furthermore, it can still be consulted to advantage, and the illustrations have not been surpassed for accuracy, beauty, and value in demonstrating the process of embryological development within the uterus, together with the relative association of the adjacent organs.

William Hunter has himself outlined the circumstances in which he embarked on the venture, which are best described in his own words, but the date he gives, 1751, is erroneous, as the captions to the plates and the dates on the drawings suggest 1750:

ANATOMIA
UTERI HUMANI GRAVIDI
TABULIS ILLUSTRATA,

AUCTORE

GULIELMO HUNTER,

SERENISSIMAE REGINAE CHARLOTTAE MEDICO EXTRAORDINARIO,
IN ACADEMIA REGALI ANATOMIAE PROFESSORE,
ET SOCIETATUM, REGIAE ET ANTIQUARIAE, SOCIO.

BIRMINGHAMIAE EXCUDEBAT JOANNES BASKERVILLE, MDCCLXXIV.

LONDINI PROSTANT APUD S. BAKER, T. CADELL, D. WILSON, G. NICOL, ET J. MURRAY.

THE ANATOMY
OF THE
HUMAN GRAVID UTERUS
EXHIBITED IN FIGURES,

BY

WILLIAM HUNTER,

PHYSICIAN EXTRAORDINARY TO THE QUEEN, PROFESSOR OF ANATOMY IN THE ROYAL ACADEMY, AND FELLOW OF THE ROYAL AND ANTIQUARIAN SOCIETIES.

PRINTED AT *BIRMINGHAM* BY *JOHN BASKERVILLE*, 1774.

SOLD IN *LONDON* BY S. *BAKER* AND G. *LEIGH*, IN *York-Street*; *T. CADELL* IN THE *Strand*; D. *WILSON* AND G. *NICOL*, OPPOSITE *York-Buildings*; AND *J. MURRAY*, IN *Fleet-Street*.

Plate 5 Title-page of William Hunter's *Gravid uterus*, 1774.

"With respect to the present undertaking, in the year 1751 (*sic.* 1750) the author met with the first favourable opportunity of examining, in the human species, what before he had been studying in brutes. A woman died suddenly, when very near the end of her pregnancy, the body was procured before any sensible putrefaction had begun; the season of the year was favourable to dissection; the injection of the blood-vessels proved successful; a very able painter, in this way, was found; every part was examined in the most public manner, and the truth was thereby well authenticated.

In the course of some months, the drawings of the first ten plates were finished, and from time to time the subject was publicly exhibited, with such remarks as had occurred in the examination of the several parts. Many lovers of this study approved of the author's proposal to publish the anatomy of the gravid uterus, illustrated by those ten plates: the work was immediately put into the hands of our best artists; and subscriptions were received. In the mean time a second subject was procured; which, though the weather happened to be unfavourable afforded a few supplemental figures of importance enough to be taken into the work. And before the engravings were finished, a third subject occurred very opportunely, which cleared up some difficulties, and furnished some useful additional figures.

The original plan having been only to publish the first ten plates, as a ground work for farther improvements in this branch of anatomy, to be added whenever good opportunities should be offered, the author now began to entertain hopes of being able to give a much more compleat work. He foresaw that, in the course of some years, by diligence, he might procure in this great city, so many opportunities of studying the gravid uterus, as to be enabled to make up a tolerable system; and to exhibit, by figures, all the principal changes that happen in the nine months of uterogestation. The execution of it has indeed taken up more time than what was at first expected: that the delay of publication has contributed not a little to the value of the work. . .

The additional expence of Mr. Baskerville's art was not incurred for the sake of elegance alone; but principally for the advantage of his paper and ink, which renders a leaf of his Press-Work an excellent preservative of the plates between which it is placed.

If it be allowed that the author has spared neither labour, nor time, nor expence in improving an important part of anatomy, this is all the merit which he can claim. In most of the dissections he was assisted by his brother Mr. John Hunter, whose accuracy in anatomical researches is so

> well known, that to omit this opportunity of thanking him for that assistance, would be in some measure to disregard the future reputation of the work itself. He owes likewise much to the ingenious artists who made the drawings and engravings; and particularly to Mr. Strange, not only for having by his own hand secured a sort of immortality to two of his plates, but for having given his advice and assistance in every part with a steady and disinterested friendship."

As early as October 1751 Hunter was advertising the set of drawings, stating that terms of subscription would be published later, and in the following year he announced that subscriptions would be taken at Mr. Millar's, a bookseller in the Strand, and at his own house in the Little Piazza, Covent Garden, where a specimen plate by Strange could be seen. He also rather prematurely announced in September 1753 that the first payment could be made, and in letters to William Cullen he also made several references to the book. On 22 February 1752, he wrote:

> "In two or three weeks I shall shew one plate finished as a specimen of the figures of the Gravid Uterus. As a piece of painting, I believe it will be the finest anatomical figure that ever was done. So it may; it will cost me a devilish deal of money. I may be allowed to speak well of the drawing and graving, you know; no merit thence in me." (Thomson, 1859, volume 1, pp. 543–4).

On 3 August 1754, he wrote:

> "Some very late occasions have increased the number of plates of the Gravid Uterus; but though that will retard the publication, the work will be much more complete for them." (*Ibid.,* p. 546).

The next information on the matter is contained in a letter dated 26 February 1765:

> "Mr. Strange has brought me proofs of four plates of my Gravid Uterus, which have been engraved at Paris so well, that I believe I shall send some more there; five are now in hand in London. They will make above thirty folio plates, and upon the whole I think a more complete work of the kind than could have been expected." (*Ibid.,* p. 554).

Three years later a letter dated 1768 reads:

> "I shall go into it in June (his new house in Windmill Street) and hope to print off my plates of the Gravid Uterus there, in the course of this summer. I shall have a printing press of my own. The engraving is now finished, only the letters of reference and the inscription at the bottom of the plates to be put in. They make thirty-four large plates. It will make a very considerable work for expence and show. Perhaps it will be the most considerable in that way that will ever be

published, so few men can have the same opportunities or better than I have had." (*Ibid.,* p. 555).

There must have been snags in the arrangements to set up a printing press in his own house (as his brother John later did), and William Hunter must also have experienced difficulty in finding an alternative printer capable of meeting his rigid requirements. Six years later he wrote to Cullen on 7 December 1774:

"Dear Sir,

Four copies of the very first impressions of the Gravid Uterus will come to your hand about the time you will receive this, sealed up and directed by my own hand to you. I beg of you to honour me by putting one of them in your own library, and one, with my best respects in the University library. The other two you will please to dispose of, as the enclosed directs, one for Dr. Baillie, and one for the University Library at Glasgow, which you will be so good as to deliver to them with my affection.

If the examination of this work were to give you a little pleasure, I think it would be a very affecting pleasure to you, who knows that but for you, I should never, in all probability, have known anything of the matter. (The letter continues to suggest that if it had not been dedicated to the King, it would have been dedicated to William Cullen.)" (*Ibid.,* p. 556).

Hunter had intended to supplement his atlas by publishing a separate text on the anatomy of the gravid uterus, and he left an uncompleted manuscript on the subject which was published twenty years after the atlas. It was edited by Matthew Baillie, who in his introduction explained that he was not previously experienced enough to evaluate the manuscript, and to prepare it for publication. It was finally printed as *An anatomical description of the human gravid uterus and its contents,* London, 1794, and a second edition by Edward Rigby was published in 1843.

In the Hunterian Museum at Glasgow there is a portfolio (Az. 1.4) containing sixty-one drawings by Jan Van Rymsdyk for William Hunter's *Anatomy of the gravid uterus.* Some of these are rough drafts of completed drawings and others are for separate figures later grouped in the published plates. Plates I–X are from the first specimen of a woman who died in 1750 at the end of her ninth month of pregnancy. Plate I shows the abdomen opened by crucial incision, and was engraved by François Aliamet. Plate II is the same viewed from the right side, and was engraved by Louis Gerard Scotin, while Plate III, a view from the left side and downwards, was engraved by Thomas Major. Plate IV is a front view of the womb and the contents of the pelvis, engraved by Robert Strange, as was Plate VI, showing the child in the womb in a natural position. A sketch of the latter accompanies the finished drawing (Plates 6--7). It was these two engravings by (Sir) Robert Strange (1721–1792) which earned him special praise from Hunter in his preface. Plate V, a first view of the unopened womb, was engraved by Johann Sebastian Müller. Plate VII shows a front view of the cavity of the womb, the child having been removed, and was engraved by François Simon Ravenet, and Plate VIII depicts the parts behind the womb, which is folded over to the front, and was engraved by Charles Grignion (1717–1810). Plate IX is of the side view of the pelvis and contents cut down through the centre. Plate X consists of three figures, Figure 1 being of a dry specimen of the outside of the front of the womb; Figure 2 is of the inside of the placenta, removed and injected with wax; and Figure 3, which was added later, shows a portion of the internal surface of the womb of a woman who died two days after delivery. These were engraved by Charles Canot. Plates XI and XII are from William Hunter's second subject, XI being the womb of a woman who died of flooding in the ninth month, of which there are two drawings (one unused), and which was engraved by Pierre Maleuve (or Maleuvre). Plate XII shows the womb and vagina opened, and was engraved by J. Mitchel.

A specimen from a third subject in the ninth month of pregnancy is featured in Plate XIII, showing a child in the womb with buttocks presenting and head upmost. This was engraved by Mechel (possibly Mitchell or J. Mitchel). Plate XIV consists of three figures which are on separate drawings, and feature the fourth subject at nine months. Figure 1 shows the muscular fasciculi on the inside of the womb, depicting the inner surface of the posterior part. The original drawing is signed with Rymsdyk's initials and dated 9 June 1766. Figure 2 (3 on drawing) is a side view of the same womb in miniature, and Figure 3 (2 on drawing) shows the inner surface of the interior part. The plate was engraved by Menil. Plate XV consists of five figures from Hunter's fifth subject, all showing the arterial system of the pregnant womb. The engraving is by François Aliamet. All these subjects were at full term, and all the drawings were executed by Rymsdyk.

Plate XVI was drawn by Edward Edwards (1738–1806) and engraved by Michell, the drawing bearing the date 1764. It is of the sixth subject, who was eight months pregnant, and shows the womb injected and dissected. The same specimen is featured in Plates XVII–XIX, and it is interesting to note that these were drawn by Rymsdyk, so that he and Edwards had worked on the same subject, Plate XVII being a side view of the specimen in Plate XVI. It was engraved by Menil, as was Plate XVIII, showing the upper part of the womb. Plates XIX and XX were of the same specimen, and were also drawn by Rymsdyk. The first shows the front of the womb, the drawing being dated 1764,

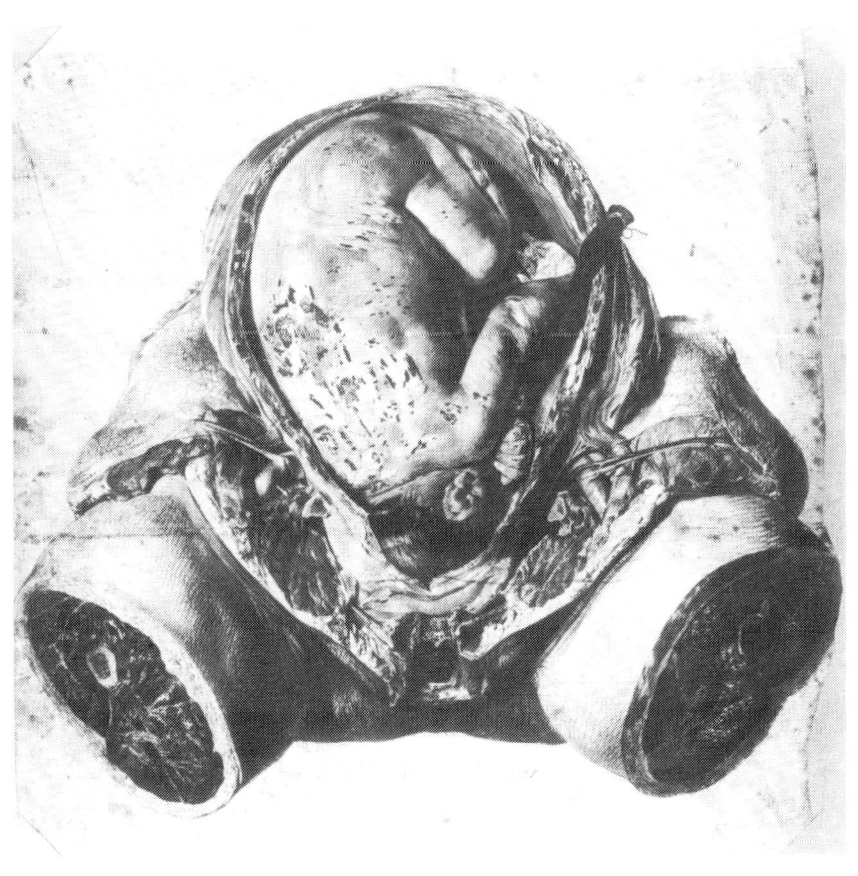

Plate 6 Rymsdyk's original drawing, dated 1750, of the fetus at term in the womb, for William Hunter's *Gravid uterus,* 1774. (Hunterian Collection, Glasgow).

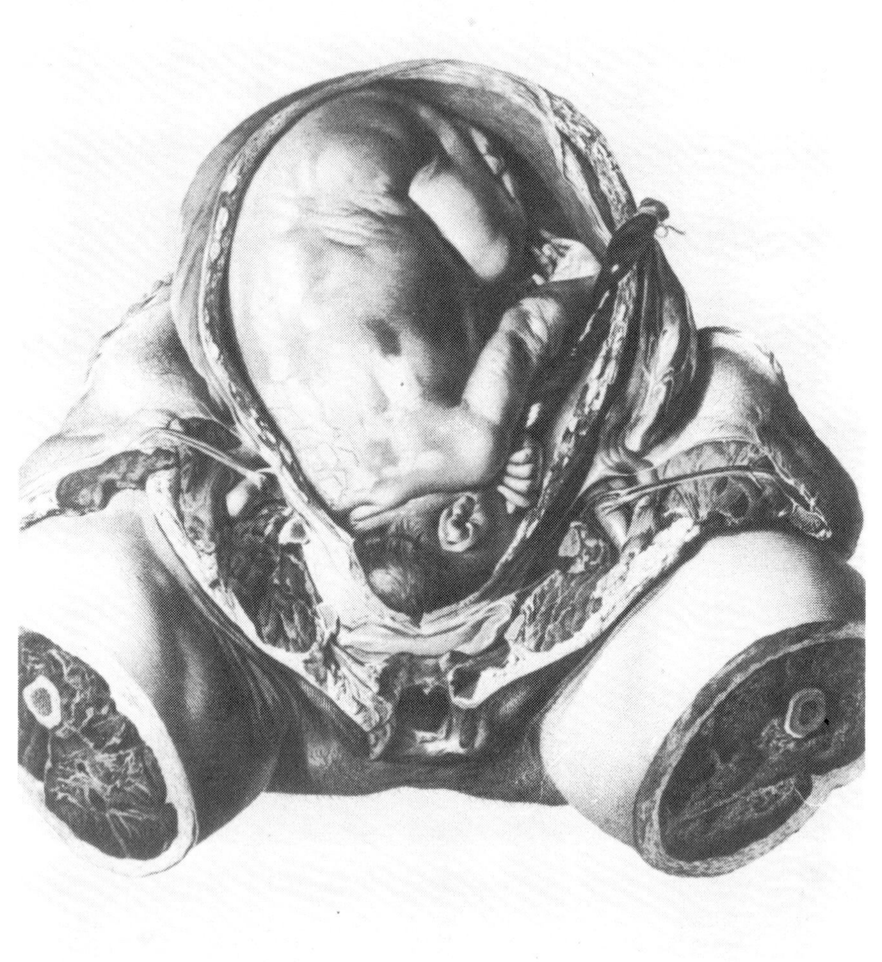

Plate 7 Engraving by Robert Strange of Rymsdyk's original drawing for William Hunter's *Gravid uterus,* 1774, Table VI.

and the engraving being by J. Fougeron. Plate XX shows the womb by Henry Bryer; this drawing also is dated 1764.

The next two plates, both engraved by François Aliamet, are of Hunter's seventh subject, at seven months, and were not from drawings by Rymsdyk; they complete the trio for which he was not responsible. Plate XXI is of the womb opened by crucial incision, the adjacent parts being shown in outline. It was drawn by Alexander Cozens, who was drawing master at Christ's Hospital from 1749–1754. The drawing for Hunter has been described by Arthur S. Marks (1967) in an article which provides additional information on Cozens and his association with Hunter's book. Plate XXII shows the contents of the pelvis, and was drawn by Nicholas Blakey, who also drew a female fetus of about five months for Hunter in 1749. The two figures, accompanied by Hunter's manuscript, which is dated from Hatton Garden, 15 June 1749, have been reproduced by K. Bryn Thomas (1960).

Hunter's eighth subject was six months pregnant, and was featured in Plates XXIII and XXIV, the latter containing four figures for which there are separate drawings, and a fifth drawing (unused) similar to Figure 1. Plate XXIII depicts the fetus in utero, and Plate XXIV shows the placenta in Figure 1; a section of half of the placenta in Figure 2; the decidua, with convoluted uterine arteries in Figure 3; and with uterine veins in Figure 4. A ninth subject, in the fifth month, is shown in diagrammatic form in Plate XXV with the womb opened and the fetus extracted, but still attached by the cord. This was engraved by Menil (Manil on plate).

The tenth subject was also in the fifth month of pregnancy, and is featured in four figures on Plate XXVI. Figure 1 shows a retroverted womb, and the original drawing has a book covering the vagina which was not included by the engraver, the drawing being shortened (Plate 8). Figure 2 depicts the bladder cut down through the centre and opened to show the situation of the os uteri. Figure 3 shows the back view of the contents of the pelvis, and Figure 4 has the womb opened to show the secundines and their contents. This plate was engraved by François Aliamet.

Plates XXVII to XXIX are devoted to Hunter's eleventh specimen, a subject at the beginning of her fifth month of pregnancy. Figure 1 on Plate XXVII shows a back view of the womb with the vagina slit up to show the cervix and the os uteri, and Figure 2 represents the same womb fully opened, showing the decidua reflexa on the chorion (Plate 9). The plate was engraved by Charles Canot, as were Plates XXIX and XXX. Menil engraved Plate XXVIII, which contains two figures, the first of the womb turned upside down so that the weight of the contents carried them towards the fundus, while Figure 2 shows the inside of the womb after the placenta had been separated. Plate XXIX has

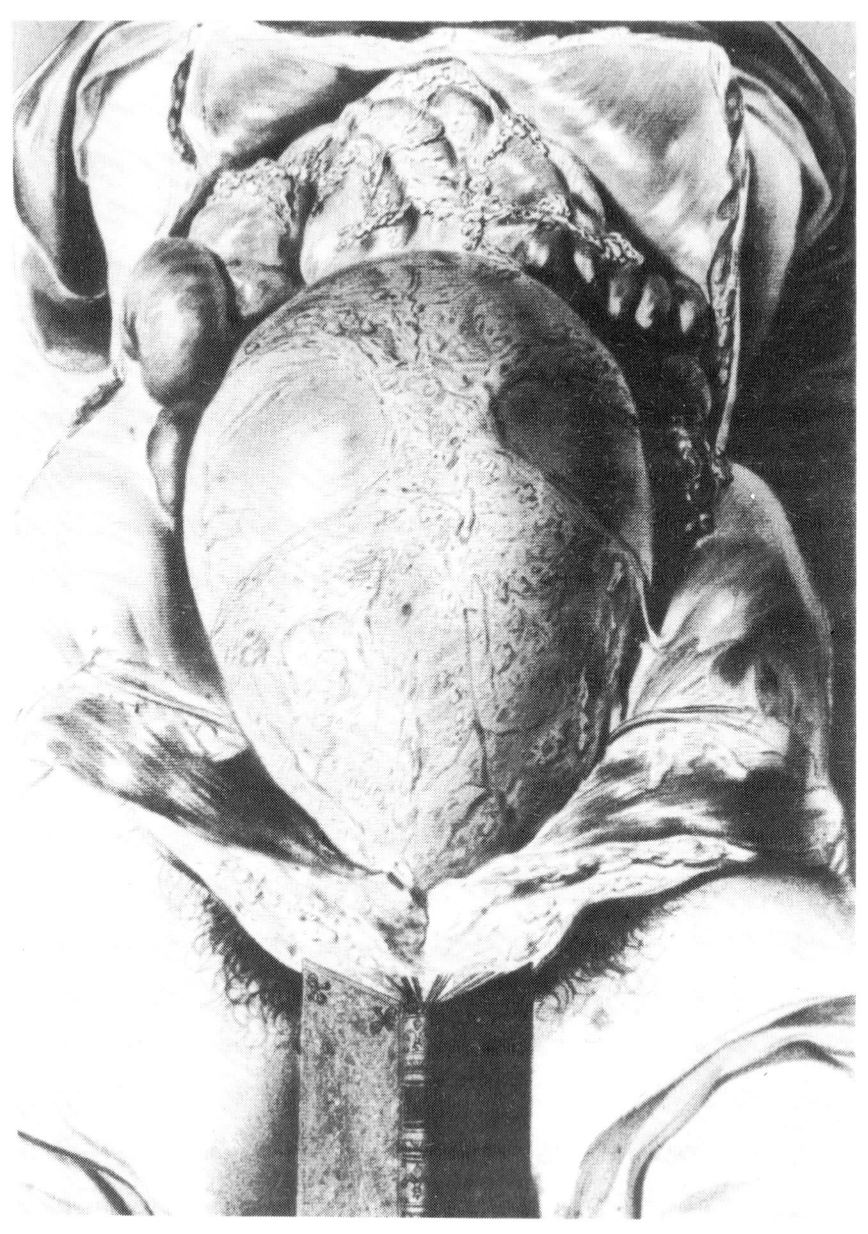

Plate 8 Rymsdyk's original drawing of retroverted womb in fifth month of pregnancy, for William Hunter's *Gravid uterus,* 1774, Table XXVI, Figure 1. The book and lower limbs are not featured in the engraving. (Hunterian Collection, Glasgow).

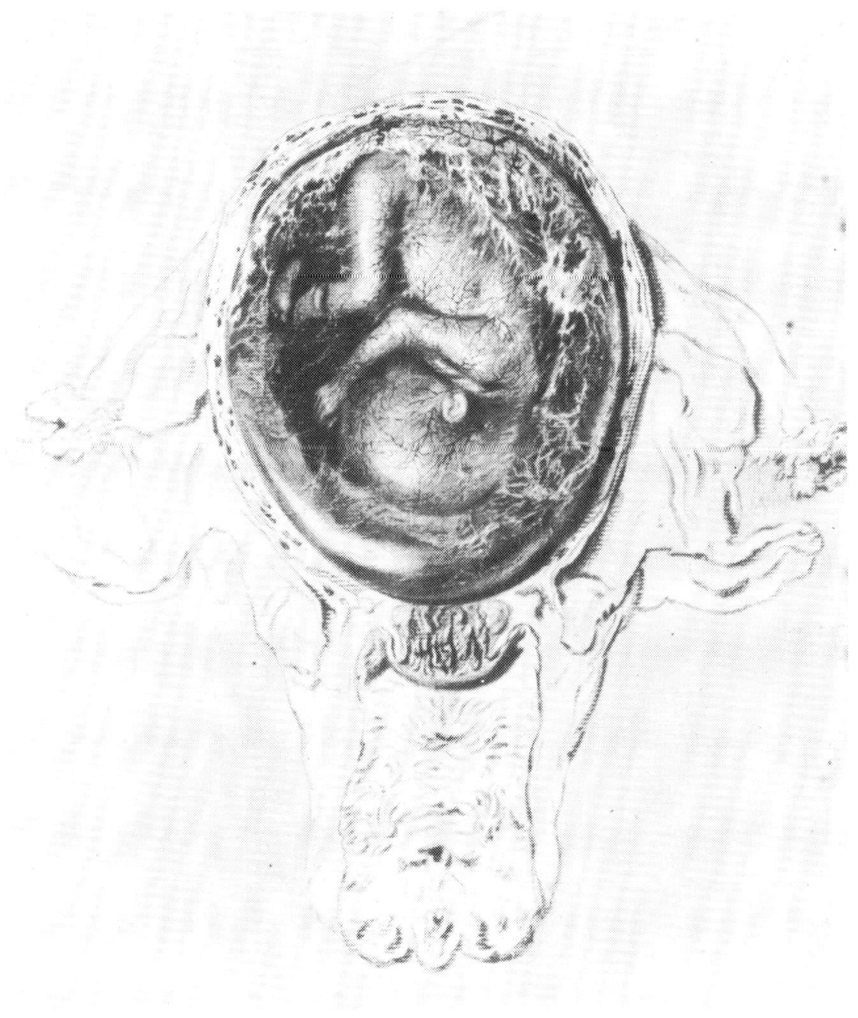

Plate 9 Rymsdyk's original drawing of a fully opened womb containing a fetus at the beginning of the fifth month of pregnancy, for William Hunter's *Gravid uterus,* 1774. This was engraved as Table XXVII, Figure II. (Hunterian Collection, Glasgow).

five figures, three being of the ovum removed from the womb, the first showing the external surface of the placenta, the second illustrating the internal surface of a portion of the decidua, considerably magnified, while Figure 3 shows a section through the ovarium and corpus luteum. Figures 4 and 5 are from another delivery, at nine months, 4 showing a portion of the decidua, and 5 part of the womb and secondines.

Hunter's twelfth subject was in the fourth month of pregnancy, and Plates XXX and XXXI are from this case. Plate XXX is of the injected womb, opened on its fore part to give a full view of the external surface of the placenta. Plate XXXI has three figures from two separate drawings. Figure 1 is a back view of the womb, opened to expose the outer surface of the decidua and the neck of the womb. Figure 2 is the same after the inverted portion of the womb had been removed, together with the decidua, to show the fetus in the liquor amnii through the transparent membranes, the other tissues being represented in diagrammatic form. Figure 3 shows the corpus luteum in the left ovary, cut through to show its cavity at this period. The engraving was by Menil.

Plate XXXII, featuring the thirteenth specimen at full three months, is of particular significance in that it was the only one engraved by the artist, Jan Van Rymsdyk. Also it is represented by eight separate drawings, as if he took special care over this specimen, and it is interesting to note that Figure 1 is represented by drawings in which the fetus is facing left (as in the engraving), and also right. Perhaps it is also significant that Rymsdyk not only did not engrave any of the other plates, but also that he did not engrave those for his own book, *Museum Britannicum.* Figure 1 is a front view of the womb opened to show the fetus and the cervix uteri, and there are two separate diagrammatic drawings of this. Figure 2 shows a longitudinal section of the womb, placenta and membranes, the fetus being removed, but still attached by the cord. There are two drawings of this, and also of the diagrammatic drawing which is engraved as part of Figure 2.

Abortions are the subject of the six figures constituting Plate XXXIII, which are all accompanied by diagrammatic representations on the plate. Figures 1 and 2 illustrate an abortion of about nine weeks, the second being a section; Figures 3 and 4 are of an abortion of about eight weeks, the latter showing the decidua opened by crucial incision; and Figures 5 and 6 are also of the same period of gestation, one consisting only of the chorion, and the other showing it opened to display the fetus. This plate was engraved by Thomas Worlidge.

Plate XXXIV was engraved by George Powle, and consists of nine figures representing conceptions at very early stages of development. Figures 1 and 2 are supposed to be about five weeks, and Figures 3 and 4 are in the fourth week. Figure 5 and 6 are dated at about three weeks, and the original drawings are dated 9 and 10 November 1770 respectively. There is a separate preliminary drawing for Figure 5 signed J.V.R. and dated 20 July 1769. Figure 7 is of a more advanced state of a supposed conception in the womb, and Figures 8 and 9 are of supposed conceptions, showing that the projection of the chorion into the cavity of the decidua is less in proportion as the conception is younger.

In addition to Rymsdyk, three other artists were involved in the drawings, each responsible for one, but there were at least sixteen engravers employed in producing the thirty-four plates. The work must have cost Hunter a considerable sum of money, and in manuscript copies of his lectures he mentions: "One of them cost 65 guineas, another 45 guineas, another 100 guineas." (Edward A. Schumann, 1940–41, p. 182; and Royal College of Surgeons, 42. c. 30, folio 242 verso). These sums are extremely high for that period, and it is not clear if these were paid to the artist, engraver, or included the entire cost of producing the plates. We have no record of money paid to Rymsdyk except for one item found by Helen Brock (personal communication, 3 November 1978): "I have worked through William Hunter's bank account at Drummonds branch of the Royal Bank of Scotland at Charing Cross. I could find only one record of a payment to Rymsdyk. £20.0.0. in 1766. Presumably other times Hunter paid him in cash."

William Hunter had mentioned in a letter to Cullen that he intended to publish the atlas from his own premises, but either he experienced difficulties in setting up a press there, or his ambitious project for an elephant folio size volume prompted him to engage an experienced, well-established printer of repute who could cope with the problems not only of size, but of special paper and ink. Hunter was a keen book collector, and particularly interested in the early printers and their choice of founts. He left an unfinished manuscript on the history of printing (Illingworth, 1971). John Baskerville (1706–1775) of Birmingham had produced several editions of the classics, and was a first-class craftsman. Hunter was a perfectionist, and obviously wanted the outstanding printer of the period to print the results of the efforts of the best artists and engravers, who had faithfully reproduced the dissections executed by William Hunter and his brother John, to whom he acknowledged his gratitude, and who was probably responsible for most of the anatomical work.

The pages of the book originally measured 22 x 16½ inches, and the title-page has the title printed in both Latin and English. The textual description opposite the plates are also in both languages. It was priced at six guineas, but a year after his death, and ten years after publication, copies were offered at 3½ guineas. Several later editions were issued, including one in 1815 with a preface by Thomas Denman, and in 1818 the Baskerville sheets were reissued in what became known as the Ballantyne edition, with a frontispiece portrait of John

Haighton. The portrait is dated 1818, the title-page is still dated 1774, but the plates are dated 1815. An undated edition was published in London by Edward Lumley at five guineas, and in 1851 the Sydenham Society printed an edition in which the plates were lithographed from the original copper-plates. The plates were also reproduced in several other publications.

Hunter's *Gravid uterus* was not only an elegantly produced pictorial atlas for teaching obstetrics: it made significant contributions to both obstetrics and embryology. Scott, Hunt and Keys (1964) include among William Hunter's original observations, proof that the placenta has a twofold circulation; the first description of the round ligament; the naming of the linea alba; and proof that lymphatics are not continuous with the blood vessels. In a paper on "The great anatomical atlases", K. Bryn Thomas (1974) wrote: ". . . the great anatomical atlases began with Vesalius in 1543 and ended with William Hunter in 1774", and most students of the subject will be in complete agreement with that statement.

The original drawings, some plaster of Paris casts, and many of the final dissected specimens are still preserved in the Hunterian Museum at Glasgow, so that they can be compared with those in the book. Many other drawings by Rymsdyk are housed there, and some have been roughly classified by Helen Brock (personal communication, 2 August 1979) as Abnormal fetuses and monsters (15); Diseased organs (57); Bones and joints, diseased and normal (17); Male reproductive system (6); Gravid uterus, diseased and normal, unpublished (13); Pathology (6); together with some of the original drawings for *Medical Observations and Inquiries* and other periodicals, and some comparative anatomy drawings. Many of these require the expert knowledge of anatomists and pathologists to identify them, to link them up with any existing specimens, and possibly with published illustrations. This presents a further problem because many engravings do not carry the names of the artists, and many of the original drawings are unsigned. Some of the drawings illustrate articles communicated by Hunter, but not written by him, and many other subjects were commissioned by him for publications which he did not live to complete. Drawings by Rymsdyk which have been identified in publications include the following:

Three plates engraved by J. Miller to illustrate William Hunter's "The history of an aneurysm of the aorta, with some remarks on aneurysms in general" (*Medical Observations and Inquiries,* 1, 1757, pp. 323–357). Four plates, also engraved by Miller, to "A singular case of the separation of the ossa pubis", communicated by Hunter, with "Remarks on the symphysis of the ossa pubis", by William Hunter (pp. 333–339). (*Ibid.,* 2, 1762, pp. 321–339, with explanations of the plates on pp. 415–418). Plate I contains five figures, Plate

III, three figures and Plate IV, two figures. Hunter's "Observations on the bones, commonly supposed to be elephant bones, which have been found near the River Ohio in America" (*Philosophical Transactions,* 58, 1768, pp. 34–45, with Plate 4). This contains six figures from three original drawings by Rymsdyk, three drawn from specimens in the British Museum, and the others from material in John Hunter's collection. All the original drawings are in Glasgow.

Three drawings by Rymsdyk of the pelvis of a dwarf who was the subject of caesarean section have been regarded in medical history as recording the first case of a person with rickets undergoing this operation. Martha Rhodes, a dwarf of about four foot four inches, aged twenty-three years, was operated on by Henry Thomson assisted by John Hunter. This was described in "A case of the caesarean section, by William Cooper, communicated by Dr. Hunter. Read 1769" (*Medical Observations and Inquiries,* 4, 1771, pp. 261–271). It was followed by "An account of the performing of the caesarean operation, with remarks by Henry Thomson, communicated by Dr. Hunter" (pp. 272–287). Plates II and III, and Figure 1 on Plate IV illustrate both communications, these plates with separately-paged captions being at the end of the volume. Martha Rhodes (named as Mary in Thomson's account), died a few hours after the operation, and the child, born with an excrescence over is nose, died two days later.

William Hunter's quarrel with his brother John over priority respecting the structure and function of the placenta and the decidua, and with others on various other matters, are not of concern to us in this study. This, and other events in his active life are recorded by Teacher (1900), and await fuller investigation in the Hunterian Collection at Glasgow. In 1770 he moved to his purpose-built premises in Great Windmill Street with its dissecting room, lecture theatre and museum housing objects of art, archaeology, geology, mineralogy and natural history. He died on 30 March 1783, leaving it, with £8,000, to Glasgow University, on condition that it remained in London for thirty years for the use of his partner William Cruikshank (1745–1800) and his nephew Matthew Baillie (1761–1823). In 1802 Baillie informed Glasgow University that they could have the museum when they had a building suitable to house it, which was in 1807, although it was not finally installed there until two years later.

William Hunter had not included his brother John in his Will, and left Long Calderwood, their birthplace, to Matthew Baillie, who immediately gave it to John. It later reverted to Baillie.

In 1772 Jan Van Rymsdyk made his final drawing for a figure on Plate XXXIV of William Hunter's *Gravid uterus,* and this was probably intended to be his last medical drawing. In that year he started work on his *Museum Britannicum,* and applied to the British Museum for permission to copy specimens there. In that book (see Chapter 6) he revealed more of his personal life than has been discovered elsewhere, and also revealed his animosity towards William Hunter. While drawing for William, Rymsdyk was performing a similar service for John Hunter, and we suggest that he had a closer affinity with the younger brother, sharing a common interest in natural history, and probably mixing with a class of person nearer Rymsdyk's own social environment.

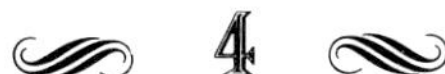

RYMSDYK'S DRAWINGS FOR JOHN HUNTER (1728–1793)

"One of the best artists whom Hunter employed was Jan Van Rymsdyk."
William LeFanu.

While making drawings for William Hunter, Rymsdyk was simultaneously working for William Smellie and C. N. Jenty. He also made the drawings still preserved in John Hunter's collection at the Royal College of Surgeons of England, but it is probable that these were executed mainly between 1755 and 1760, while John was still working with his brother, although a few are dated as late as 1765. Many of the drawings were not published until many years later, others were not used during Hunter's lifetime, and since many of the drawings were not signed or dated, their attribution has been difficult. A brief survey of Hunter's career, with particular reference to his activities while Rymsdyk was alive, will throw some light on the problems involved, and on the association between the two men.

The life of John Hunter has been chronicled more exhaustively than that of his brother, and he has been the subject of several biographical studies, numerous Hunterian Orations, and many articles covering various aspects of his career. Brief biographies were appended to some of his posthumous publications (as noted later), and more recent books include studies by George C. Peachey (1924), S. Roodhouse Gloyne (1950), and Jessie Dobson (1969). John Hunter was a careful investigator, an original thinker, and a stimulator of thought in others, as evidenced in his letters to Edward Jenner (1749–1823), thirty-two of which are preserved at the Royal College of Surgeons, and which were transcribed in *Letters from the past. From John Hunter to Edward Jenner,* 1976, edited by Eustace H. Cornelius and A. J. Harding Rains. These emphasize his eclectic interest in nature and in everything that had life. He was responsible for placing surgery on a scientific basis, and his contributions to anatomy, physiology and zoology were particularly noteworthy.

John Hunter was born at Long Calderwood, East Kilbride, near Glasgow on 13 February 1728, the youngest of a family of ten. He had little formal education, and no interest in books, but enjoyed country activities such as sport and natural history. When about seventeen he went to stay in Glasgow with his sister, whose husband was a cabinet-maker, and John assisted him. In 1748 John Hunter came to London on horseback to assist his brother William with dissection, at which he became adept. From 1749–50 he attended the classes of William Cheselden (1688–1752) at Chelsea Hospital, and in 1751 those of Percivall Pott (1714–1788), Surgeon to St. Bartholomew's Hospital. In 1754 he became a surgeon's pupil at St. George's Hospital, and William Hunter sent John to Oxford in 1755 in an attempt to improve his education and possibly acquire the polish of a gentleman, but John returned to London after a very brief period.

Resuming work with his brother, John Hunter launched himself into a period of activity in the dissecting room, and during the next four years he traced the descent of the testes in the fetus, the placental circulation, the nasal and olfactory nerves, and also the lymphatic system. In 1759 he suffered from inflammation of the lungs, probably as the result of many hours spent in the dissecting room, and the following year he joined the services as an Army Surgeon. He sailed for Belle Isle in 1761, and saw active service there and in Portugal, where he also found time to study local natural history and geology. During this time he also investigated the coagulation of the blood, gunshot wounds, and inflammation.

In May 1763 John Hunter returned to England, bringing with him much material resulting from his observations. His position in William's anatomy school was no longer vacant, and he started in practice as a surgeon in Golden Square. He also began taking pupils in anatomy and operative surgery, but he was a poor lecturer and acquired few pupils. However, he bought two acres of land at Earl's Court and built a house. providing also facilities for dissection and maceration. There he kept many live animals, including bees and leopards. He made his first communication to the Royal Society in 1766, and was elected a Fellow the following year, when he also became a member of the Surgeons' Corporation. John Hunter was elected Surgeon to St. George's Hospital in 1768 and moved to the house in Jermyn Street which had been vacated by William. There he had house pupils and apprentices, including Edward Jenner, and later Everard Home, whose sister Anne he married in 1771.

The first publication in book form by John Hunter was *The natural history of the human teeth,* 1771, with a second part entitled *A practical treatise on the diseases of the teeth,* 1778, the two parts appearing in a second edition in the same year, and a third in 1803. The "advertisement" or preface states that most of the observations in the book were made by the author before 1755, that "the substance of them (was) constantly demonstrated after that period, in Dr. Hunter's course of anatomical lectures. The figures were drawn by Mr. Rymsdyk, under the author's direction, and engraved by Mess. Strange, Grignion, Ryland, and others."

This was when John was still working with his brother William ("Dr. Hunter"), and before John went to Portugal. The book contains sixteen plates, some of them consisting of several figures. These range from complete skulls and jaws, to individual teeth and sections thereof. Plate VII is the only one bearing the name "J. Van Riemsdyk" engraved as part of the plate which depicts "the bones of the head of a very old woman, who had lost her teeth a considerable time before death." There are twenty-six original drawings at the Royal College of Surgeons; they are mounted on thirteen separate leaves in the portfolio (II, pp. 184–192) (Plates 10–11).

In 1773 John Hunter began giving lectures on the theory and practice of surgery to his apprentices, and to others paying fees, but in the same year he suffered his first attack of angina pectoris. Four years later, after suffering from vertigo, he visited Bath, where he met Jenner, who diagnosed that Hunter had an organic affection of the heart, which eventually led to his sudden death while attending a meeting at St. George's Hospital on 16 October 1793.

For this particular purpose we are not concerned with John Hunter's activities after Rymsdyk ceased to be associated with him as an artist. This is particularly difficult to determine since few of the original drawings are dated, and some of them were not published until many years after they were made. Some were used to illustrate papers published in the *Philosophical Transactions,* and certain of these were later reprinted in *Observations on certain parts of the animal oeconomy,* 1786, and in his *Works,* 1835 to 1837. However, the last dated original drawing by Rymsdyk is 1765. John Hunter had a great appreciation of the work performed by artists, and it is recorded that he "never took fees from curates, authors, or artists." In 1775 he engaged William Bell to make anatomical preparations and drawings, and to superintend the museum. He lived as a member of Hunter's extensive household, which makes one speculate on whether Jan Van Rymsdyk ever lived in the households of John or William Hunter. Bell stayed there until 1789, when he joined the East India Company, went abroad, and died in 1792.

John Hunter employed several other artists, including J. St. Aubin, who trained William Clift (1775–1849), the most important figure in the history of the Hunterian Museum, and who was largely responsible for its survival after the death of Hunter. Jessie Dobson (1959) has provided some information on

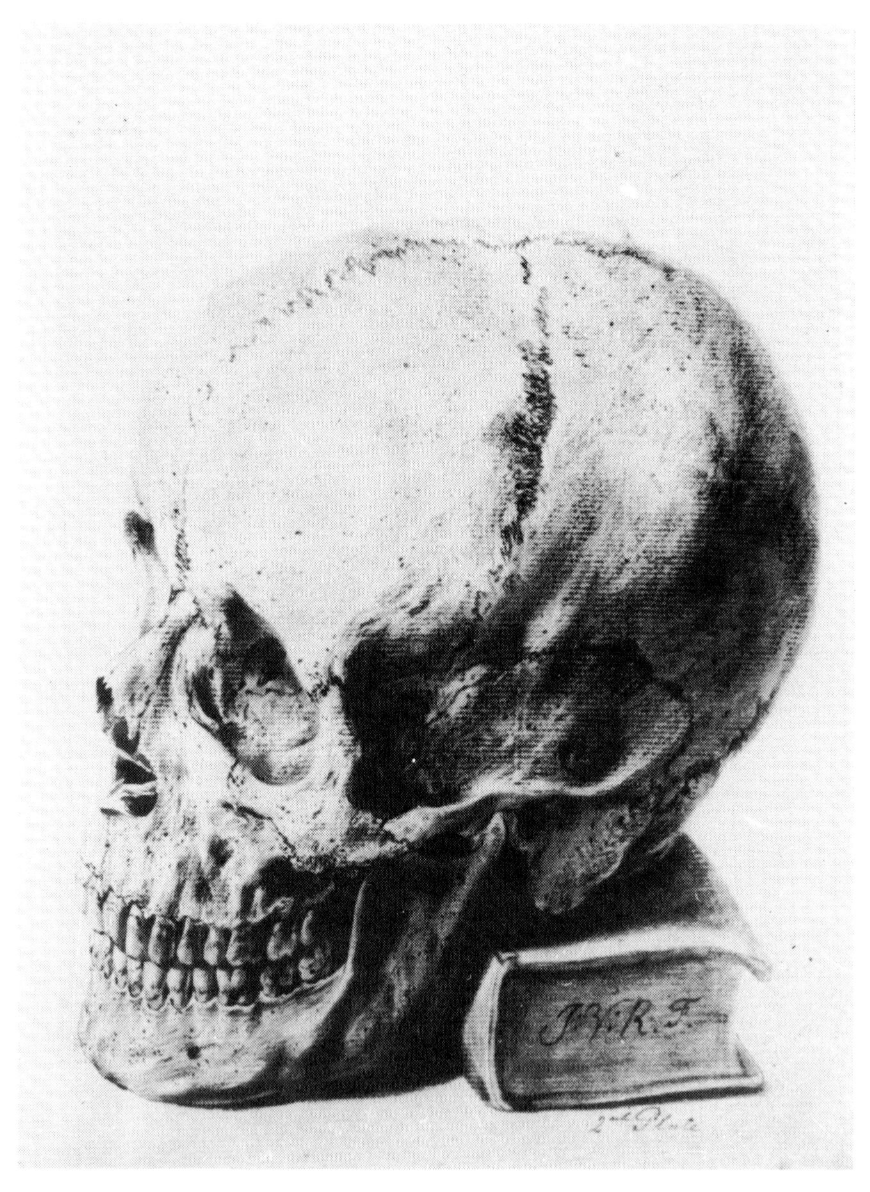

Plate 10 Rymsdyk's original drawing of skull for Plate III, Figure 2 of John Hunter's *Natural history of the human teeth,* 1771. The lower half only was engraved, and the initials on the end of the book were omitted. (Royal College of Surgeons of England).

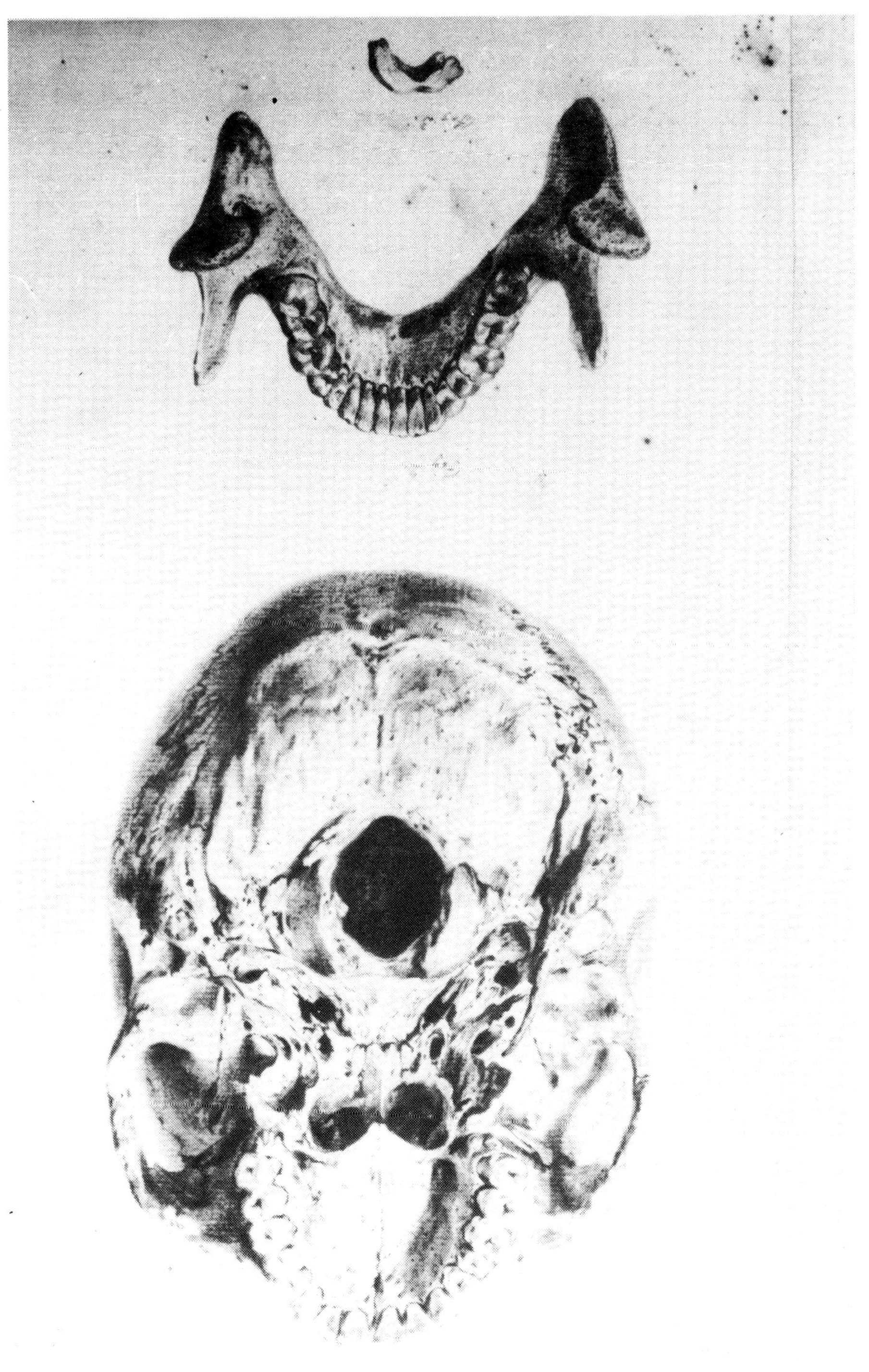

Plate 11 Rymsdyk's original drawings for Plate IV, Figures 1 and 2 of John Hunter's *Natural history of the human teeth,* 1771. Only the upper half of the top figure was engraved. (Royal College of Surgeons of England).

these artists. William LeFanu (1978) describes their work, and records other important collections of natural history drawings acquired by Hunter.

In 1786 two books by John Hunter were published, both printed in his own house in Castle Street: *A treatise on the venereal disease,* and *Observations on certain parts of the animal oeconomy.* The latter contains the following: "A description of the situation of the testis in the foetus, with its descent into the scrotum", with five plates from drawings by Rymsdyk; "Observations on the glands situated between the rectum and the bladder, called vesiculae seminales", with one plate drawn by Rymsdyk; followed by nine papers from the *Philosophical Transactions,* with one plate (II) by Rymsdyk, who also contributed the two plates illustrating "A description of the nerves which supply the organ of smelling." A second edition of this book was published in 1792, with additional reprints of papers from the *Philosophical Transactions,* but these were not illustrated by Rymsdyk. All these illustrations were reproduced in the separate volume of plates published with Hunter's *Works,* 1837. Many of the plates do not bear the name of the artist, and numerous original drawings in the portfolios containing Rymsdyk's contributions are likewise unidentified, so that it has been impossible positively to attribute their authorship. We do know that Hunterian Drawings II.F. contains the entire series for the book on the teeth, in a bright terracotta wash, sometimes described as the "sanguine technique." Most have pencil outline drawings pasted in on the opposite page, and one has the pencil outline only, with the note: "This drawing is missing. Mr. Grinion (sic) has it". Hunterian Drawings III.S contains seventeen miscellaneous drawings identified as by Rymsdyk, two being of the head of a child without a cranium, the drawing being signed and dated 1 January 1755. An annotation to this reads:

> "A drawing of a monstrous Child that was born without any Cranaum, had only a bag that lay on the Bases of the skull, the true skin all round where it terminated was puckered in towards the Bag similar to that of a sore so that it was not like a Cranaum that had been sawed off. The skin of this Bag was very thin and contained a Gellatenous fluid."

Many of the other drawings have extensive descriptions appended, but the writing is not that of Hunter.

Pathological Drawings II.S. contains five drawings of the human uterus, one of which shows a fetus *in situ* and another of which is dated 1756. Pathological Drawings V.II. contains four drawings illustrating an aneurysm of the curvature of the spine, one being signed and dated 8 June 1765.

Hunterian Drawings IV.E also contains miscellaneous subjects, eleven of the drawings probably having been made by Rymsdyk, and several others possibly by his hand.

Some of the specimens from which these drawings were made are still in the Hunterian Museum, but many others were destroyed during World War II. Surviving Hunterian specimens have been described by Jessie Dobson (1970), who has reproduced two of Rymsdyk's drawings. Figure 16 shows the tongue and fauces of the crocodile (Drawing Book C, p. 919), and Figure 18 the tongue of a porpoise (Drawing Book C, p. 926). This Drawing Book C contains at least twenty-seven other drawings by Rymsdyk, covering a wide range of subjects. It is probable that many of the drawings were initiated by John Hunter for future use but, like his brother William, he did not survive long enough to complete his plans.

A painting of a group of animals includes a peccary, two agoutis, an ichneumon (similar to a mongoose), and a chough (or red-legged crow), is in oil on canvas. It is unsigned, but William Clift noted, "said to have been painted by J. V. Rymsdyk". This is an unusual grouping of animals by Rymsdyk, and is certainly not in the same class as the paintings by Stubbs executed for John Hunter.

Two framed drawings by Rymsdyk of the development of the chick within the hen's egg, showing twenty-four stages, hang in the Hunterian Museum (Plates 12–13). Rymsdyk apparently made copies of these when John Hunter was preparing a collection of specimens to be housed at Kew Observatory, which was opened in 1769. These were used in the instruction of the children of George III and Queen Charlotte. When the contents of the museum were dispersed in 1841, the anatomical specimens were offered to the Royal College of Surgeons, and seventy, only five of which still survive, were received by the College. The copy of the embryology of the chick series was determined to be a duplicate (actually it contained one less figure), and duplicates were thought to have been sent to King's College. However, the present location of this item has not been traced, if indeed it survives. Rymsdyk discovered later that this copy was in the Queen's collection, and thought that he should have been credited with the work. Unfortunately, in his *Museum Britannicum* (see Chapter 6) he apparently berates William Hunter for this oversight, but probably it was John Hunter who provided the Kew drawings. Jessie Dobson (1951) has given full information on the Hunter specimens at Kew Observatory and their subsequent history.

John Hunter's posthumously published writings include *A treatise on the blood, inflammation and gun-shot wounds,* 1794, which contains a short biography of Hunter by Everard Home; *The works of John Hunter, with notes. Edited by James F. Palmer,* four volumes, with a separate book of plates, and a biography by Drewry Ottley; *Memoranda on vegetation,* 1860; and *Essays and observations on natural history, anatomy, physiology, psychology and geology,*

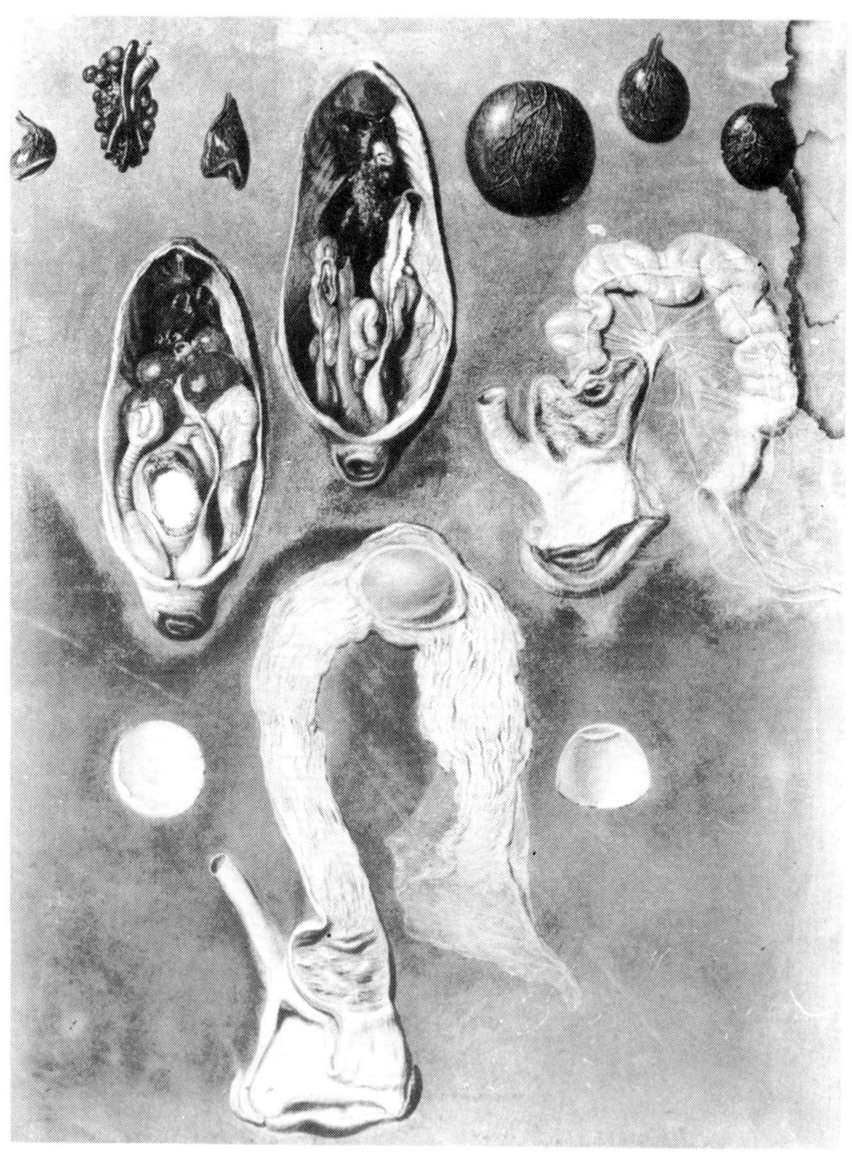

Plates 12–13 Series of drawings by Rymsdyk showing the development of the chick. These are in colour, and the two framed pictures hang in the Hunterian Museum. (Royal College of Surgeons of England).

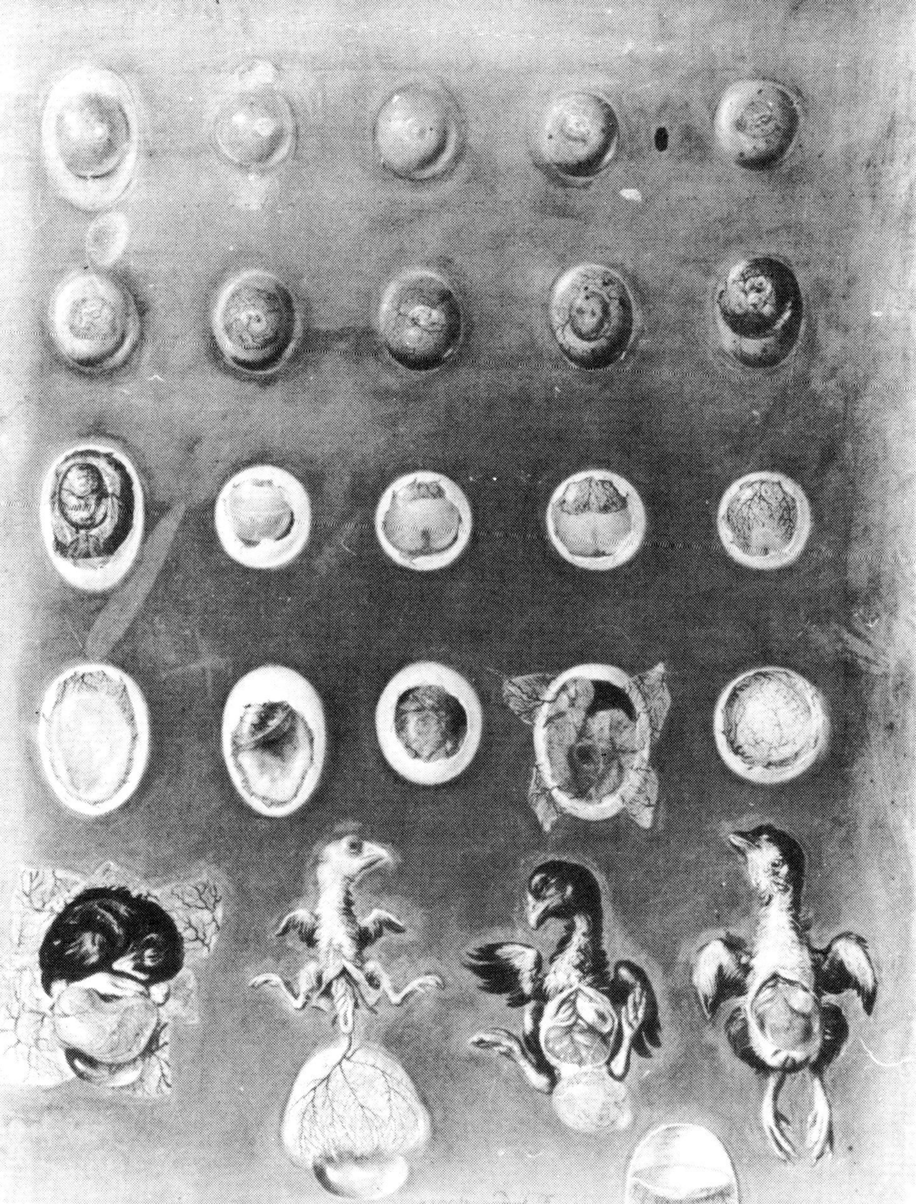

two volumes, 1861, which was edited by Richard Owen. Several of his books were translated into other languages, and appeared in numerous editions. William LeFanu (1946) has published a preliminary check-list of these, and Jessie Dobson's *John Hunter* (1969, pp. vii–xi) has a "Chronological list of John Hunter's writings". His museum was bought by the government and presented to the Royal College of Surgeons, but suffered severe damage during an air-raid in May 1941. In 1823 Everard Home burned many of John Hunter's papers, but William Clift had made copies of some of these, and was aware that Home had published a great deal of Hunter's work under his own name. The destruction of these manuscripts has been recorded in some detail by Jane M. Oppenheimer (1946).

We have noted that several of Hunter's books were printed on his own premises in Castle Street, and A. H. T. Robb-Smith (1970) has provided information on John Hunter's private press. John Richardson was the printer, and there were two pressmen. The sheets were folded and stitched on the premises, and they were also sold from there, as well as by G. Nicol and J. Johnson. Robb-Smith gives details of the number of copies printed in the various editions, their prices and sales.

Both John Hunter's writings and those of William were greatly enhanced by the illustrations drawn by Jan Van Rymsdyk, and it is fortunate that the originals, including many which have never appeared in print, are still preserved in the Library of the Royal College of Surgeons of England.

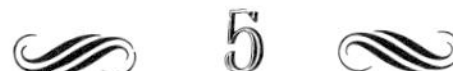

RYMSDYK'S DRAWINGS FOR CHARLES NICHOLAS JENTY

"The 'Fothergill anatomical paintings' or the 'Van Riemsdyk crayons', as they are variously called, played a basic part in early medical teaching in the United States."

Florence M. Greim.

Charles Nicholas Jenty was an elusive eighteenth-century character about whom little is known apart from his writings, and even these are rare. They seldom come on the book market, and few medical libraries possess copies. No doubt popular when first published, they were either soiled by their association with dissecting rooms, and eventually discarded, or were superseded by later publications.

Jenty probably came to London about 1745 and lectured on anatomy. He has been described as Professor of Anatomy and Surgery in London, and as "A.M.", but the dates and places of his birth and death have not been traced. Two of his books were issued from "his house in Fetter Lane", where he may have conducted his lectures, and his publications provide the only scanty clues to his origin and wanderings. Jenty's first published work was *A course of anatomico-physiological lectures on the human structure and animal oeconomy, interspersed with various critical notes extracted from memoirs, transactions of learned societies, &c. and pathological observations, deduced from the dissection of morbid bodies, (etc.)*, three volumes, London, 1757, and in the preface (p. 10) to the first volume he states:

> "Tho' I have been reading English authors for these dozen years past, and understand the language sufficiently to come at the sense, nevertheless I am conscious that these lectures are not so well penned, as if they came from an English hand."

The work was based mainly on the writings of Winslow, Haller, Ruysch, Morgagni, Monro and Heister, and contains essays on the arts of dissecting, injecting and making anatomical preparations. It made no pretence to be original, but a third edition was published in 1765. No copies of a second edition were traced by K. F. Russell (1963), who provides full bibliographical details of this and other books by Jenty (Numbered 474–484).

The octavo text volume of Jenty's *The demonstration of a pregnant uterus of a woman at her full term, (etc.)*, London, 1757, is dedicated to the Members of the Royal Academy of Surgery at Paris, and proceeds as follows:

> "Gentlemen.
>
> Though I have not offered the first fruits of my labours to our celebrated Academy; I would not have you imagine, that because I am, at present, settled in a foreign country, have so far forgot myself, as not to remember my native place, where I received the first elements of my profession from some of your most learned Members. . . .London, 1757".

These quotations suggest that Jenty was born in France and probably received his medical education in Paris. He was probably in London from 1745 until 1762, lecturing and writing books. As a lecturer he probably encountered heavy competition from the Hunter school and other individual lecturers, and this may be why in 1762 he went as Surgeon's Mate with the British Expeditionary Force under Lord Loudoun to Portugal. John Hunter (1728–1793) went as a Surgeon with the same Force, and G. E. Gask (1936–37) and Jessie Dobson (1954) have written papers providing further information on that period, but with brief mention of Jenty. However, we can establish that when the Force returned to England in 1763, Jenty remained in Portugal "on his own affairs." He later moved from Lisbon to Madrid, where he appears to have lectured on anatomy and surgery, and also published a pamphlet on amputation in 1766. A further publication bearing his name was published as *A narrative of the trial of Thomas Pierce's styptick medicines,* London, 1767, but little further is recorded of the life and work of this remarkable man. J. G. De Lint (1916) wrote a paper on the mezzotint plates in his obstetrical atlas, and J. L. Thornton and Patricia C. Want (1978) provided some additional information which had been discovered. However, C. N. Jenty will chiefly be remembered historically for the outstanding drawings by Jan Van Rymsdyk included in Jenty's two atlases, and by the originals still existing in Pennsylvania Hospital.

Jenty first published a proposal for his anatomical tables in 1756, and the following year these were published in folio, with a smaller accompanying text bearing the title *An essay on the demonstration of the human structure, half as large as nature, in four tables, from the pictures painted after dissections, for that purpose,* London, "printed for and sold by the author at his house in Fetter-Lane, and all the eminent booksellers in Europe," 1757. A Latin version was published in the same year, and the fact that text and atlas were of different sizes has often led to their separation, although they are occasionally found bound together, either with the plates folded in half or with the text leaves mounted. The plates were drawn by Rymsdyk and engraved by Edward Fisher, two of them being dated 1756 (Plate 14). The *Bibliotheca Walleriana* (No. 5151) states that the plates were printed in colour, but the copy in the Waller Library at Uppsala is hand-coloured. In his introduction Jenty stated that he had originally intended them to be colour-printed but had decided in favour of mezzotint, and that purchasers could then have them coloured either from the original paintings or from nature. The price paid would determine the extent of their perfection.

It is strange that the number of plates was limited to four, because Rymsdyk had made many more drawings for Jenty. Some were used in his atlas of the gravid uterus, and he may have had plans for other collections of plates which never matured. Jenty's *The demonstrations of a pregnant uterus of a woman at her full term. In six tables, as large as nature. Done from pictures painted after dissections, by Mr. Riemsdyk* was also published by the author from his own house in 1757, and was re-issued in the following year. In a note to the reader, Jenty explains why mezzotint was chosen for the plates:

> "If it should be asked, Why, in these Plates, I chose Mezzotinto, instead of Engraving? I answer, that not only the difficulty and Length of time requisite to have executed these TABLES, by able persons, nor the expence, which would have been considerable, prevented my Determination to Engraving; but the Engraving itself, how well soever performed, would not have answered my intention for Colouring, so well as Mezzotinto; as this method is softer, and capable of exhibiting a nearer imitation of Nature than Engraving, as Artists themselves acknowledge that Nature may admit of light and shades, well blended and softened, but never did of a harsh outline: So it must be confessed, that these Prints may want the Smartness which Engraving might have contributed; but the Softness which they possess, may approach nearer to the Imitation of Nature, when coloured, than any engraving possibly could, merely thro' the unavoidable Delineation of the Outline.
>
> Gentlemen may have these Mezzotinto Prints, coloured after the original Pictures, of different Degrees of Perfection, according to the Price allowed to the Colourer."

A footnote states that, if encouraged by the public, Jenty would publish two more plates, but apparently this support was not forthcoming, or circumstances prevented him from fulfilling his promise.

Another reason why Jenty decided against printing in colour was probably

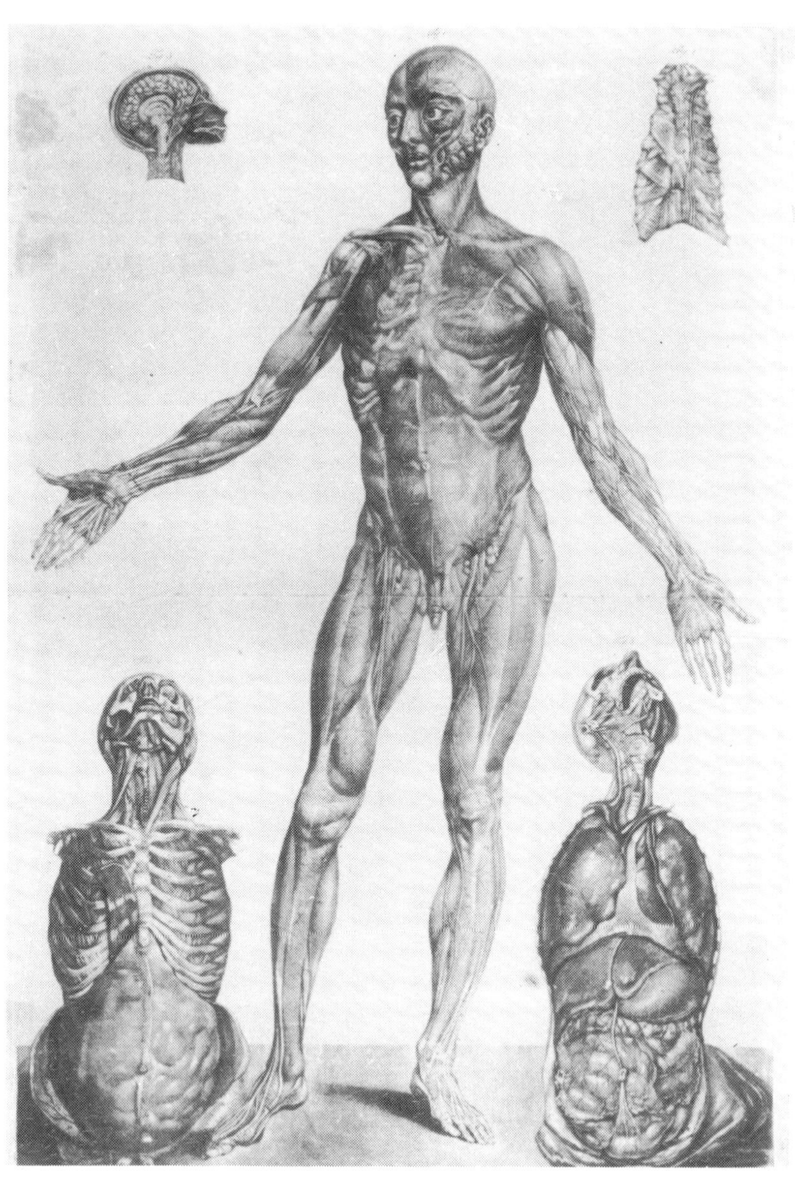

Plate 14 Mezzotint version of Rymsdyk's coloured drawing for C. N. Jenty's *Demonstration of the human structure,* 1757, Table 1.

the cost of the process and the problems involved in the production. The first anatomical illustrations to be reproduced in coloured printing were in *De lactibus sive lacteis venis,* Milan, 1627, by Gasparo Aselli (1581–1626), and consist of four folio foldout woodcuts. Black was used for the background, contours, crosshatching, veins, and for the letters engraved on the figures; dark red for the arteries, crosshatching and for shadows; and light red (or brown) for the surfaces of the intestine, the mesentery, and the liver. This involved the use of multiple blocks, and success depended on correct imposition, and the drying of the ink between processes. It is significant that in later editions the plates were engraved, and printed in black.

Coloured mezzotints were first attempted in 1704 by Jacob Christoph Le Blon (1670–1741), a native of Frankfort-on-Main, who first settled in Amsterdam as a miniature-portrait painter. He employed yellow, blue, red and probably black, but kept his process secret, although he later took out a patent for coloured copper printing. Le Blon worked in The Hague and Paris before coming about 1720, to London where he set up in business and established "The Picture Office", but became bankrupt. Returning to The Hague, and thence to Paris, he died there in 1741. Little is known about Le Blon's anatomical plates, which are very rare, but Paul Krivatsy (1968) has reproduced a previously unknown one contained in a pamphlet by Arent Cant (1695–1723), and also provides information on Le Blon and his work.

While in London, Le Blon had pupils and assistants, one of whom was Jan Ladmiral (1698–1773), who claimed Le Blon's invention as his own, and offered his services to Albinus. Six plates were published under the joint title *Anatomische voorwerpen door Jan Ladmiral* between 1736 and 1741. Two were accompanied by a text by Albinus, others illustrated preparations by Fredrik Ruysch (1638–1731), and the sixth appears to be an imitation of a plate by Le Blon dated 1721, but with no mention of Le Blon.

Jacques Fabian Gautier d'Agoty (*c.* 1717–1786) was born in Marseilles, and became an assistant to Le Blon. After the death of the latter, Gautier acquired his patent in 1745, and later claimed to be the inventor of coloured copperplate printing. His plates are impressive in size and colour, but are not outstanding anatomically, and are considered inferior to those of Ladmiral. They appear in anatomical works published mainly in Paris between 1745 and 1759, some of them being cumulations of plates from earlier publications.

These abortive attempts at the introduction of colour printing to medical subjects were not entirely successful, but were probably known to both Jenty and Rymsdyk. Jenty would have considered the cost of the venture, and Rymsdyk could not have been impressed by the artistic results, particularly if applied to his very detailed drawings.

As with the anatomical atlas, a Latin translation of *A pregnant uterus* was published simultaneously. Three of the reproductions from the drawings were by Richard Purcell, one by Edward Fisher, and two by Thomas Burgess. A German translation had the title-page printed in Latin followed by the German version, and the plates were incised by J. M. Seligman. The title-page is dated Nuremberg, 1761, but the colophon gives 1765. A Dutch translation was published some years later in Amsterdam, 1793, but in all of these are illustrations are mezzotints (Plate 15). However, in the French translation both text and plates are engraved, the latter being reduced copies of the originals, and are also reversed. This was entitled *Demonstration de la matrice d'une femme grosse et de son enfant à terme,* Paris, 1759, and Plate 1 was engraved by Danzel, the others being by Charpentier. All the drawings are ascribed to "Jean van Riemsdyk", but in fact Thomas Burgess was responsible for the drawing featured in Plate 1, as noted in the mezzotint versions. This French version was reprinted by Chereau in 1763 and 1764.

From 1755 onwards Rymsdyk made numerous drawings for Jenty, only some of which were used to these two atlases. In August 1757 Jenty presented to the Company of Surgeons "four large anatomical prints, coloured, glazed and framed", and he was invited to dine with the Company a few days later. The Company of Surgeons later became the Royal College of Surgeons of England, but it is not known if these plates were part of the property transferred to the College. Their present location has not been determined, if they have in fact survived. We are therefore unable to confirm that they were prints which were later coloured by hand. They might have been original drawings by Rymsdyk.

In a letter to James Pemberton of Philadelphia dated 7 April 1762 (Fothergill (1971), pp. 994–998), John Fothergill (1712–1780) mentioned that he was sending by Dr. Shippen a present to Pennsylvania Hospital which could be used for teaching purposes. The gift arrived in seven packing cases, and consisted of eighteen drawings framed and glazed, three gypsum casts, and skeletons of an adult and a fetus. J. A. Scott (1904) described the drawings, one of which was by Thomas Burgess, sixteen by Rymsdyk (one being signed and dated 1755), and one was of a doctor feeling the pulse of a young woman. Scott also mentioned that six of the pictures were broken in transit, but were later repaired. He provided a list of the sixteen drawings by Rymsdyk, and reproduced two of them as illustrations. Francis R. Packard (1938) reproduced two of Rymsdyk's figures, and the one by Burgess, in his history of the Pennsylvania Hospital, and Edward B. Krumbhaar (1922) reproduced the three gypsum casts and the seventeen drawings, in an article on the early history of anatomy in the United States. He also suggests (p. 285, Note 23) that one of the stages of dissection of the whole body may have been lost, but it is also

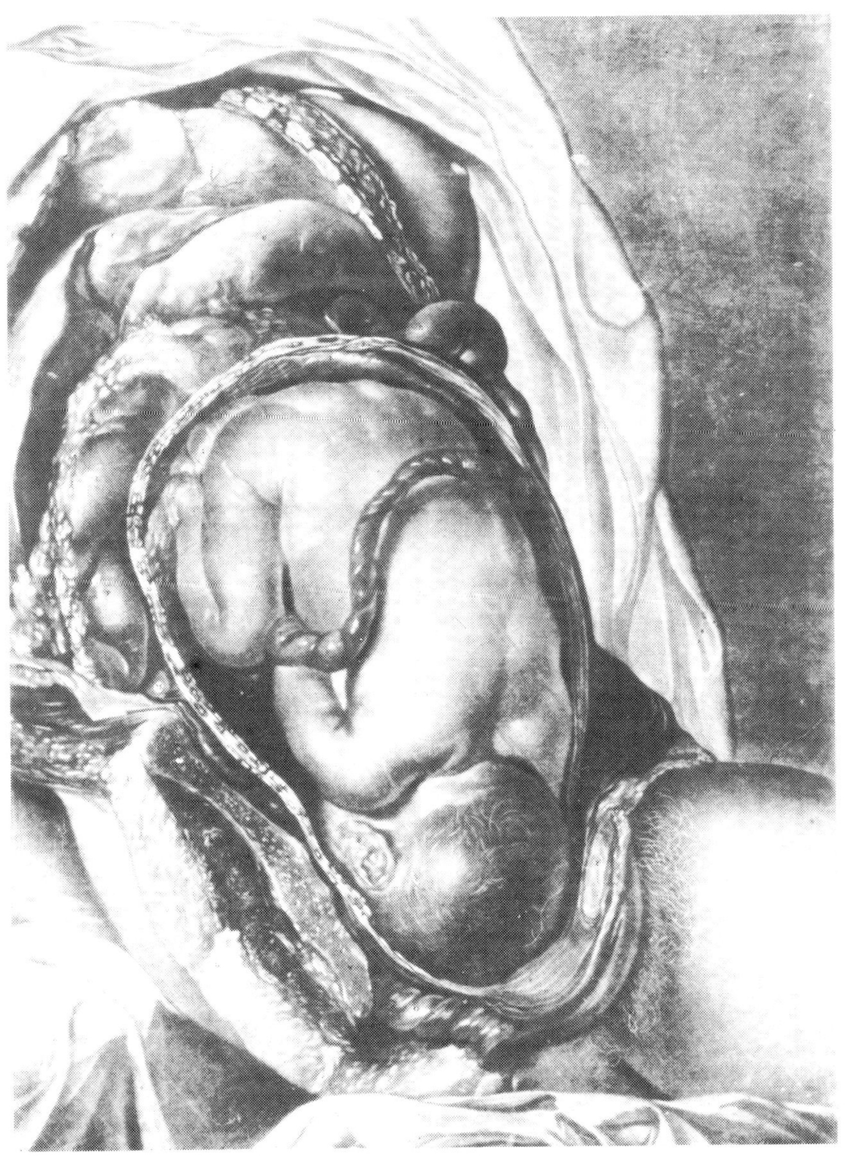

Plate 15 Mezzotint of Rymsdyk's drawings of the pregnant uterus at term, from C. N. Jenty's *Demonstrations of a pregnant uterus,* 1757, Table 4.

possible that it might have been included in the series given by Jenty to the Company of Surgeons.

All the drawings by Rymsdyk are in coloured crayons, and are still preserved in Pennsylvania Hospital. They were used by Shippen for teaching purposes, and were also exhibited to others interested, a small fee being requested. Four of the drawings (one by Burgess) were reproduced in colour in *What's New,* April 1952, and were reprinted with a foreword by Florence M. Greim (1952), who suggested that they played a basic part in medical education in the United States.

William Shippen, Jr. (1736–1808) had studied in London under the Hunters, among others, and became friendly with John Fothergill (1712–1780), who was also acquainted with Jenty. In 1762 the latter joined the British Expeditionary Force, and probably disposed of his possessions before going abroad. He certainly did not return with the Army, and possibly had already decided to remain abroad. Fothergill probably acquired the drawings, casts and skeletons direct from Jenty, and Packard (1938) suggested that the drawings cost Fothergill about two hundred guineas.

On comparing photographs of these original drawings with the atlases published by Jenty, we find that they include those for the four plates in Jenty's *Anatomical tables,* 1757, which are represented by seven drawings. These are composed of several figures, and in many of the drawings reproduced as plates, the latter differ from the former in certain details. Of the six plates in Jenty's *Gravid uterus,* (five drawn by Rymsdyk and one by Burgess), only the Rymsdyk items are among the Pennsylvania drawings. Plate 5 of this does not include the fetus, and is an example of differences between certain engraved versions and the originals. Incidentally, the Burgess drawing (Plate 1) is another surface anatomy study, while Rymsdyk's anatomical drawings are mainly of dissections, at which he excelled.

Charles Nicholas Jenty can almost be considered as a peripatetic lecturer on anatomy and surgery, although he was in London for several years, and issued most of his publications from there. We know nothing of his success as a lecturer, we have no evidence that he practised medicine, surgery or midwifery, and the only surviving evidence of his work exists in the few remaining copies of his publication, and the drawings executed for him by Jan Van Rymsdyk. These original drawings consist mainly of those displayed in Pennsylvania Hospital, and the printed versions both engraved and in mezzotint are brilliantly executed. Not fully appreciated because of their rarity, they are outstanding examples of the arts of the craftsmen, and have also ensured that Jenty's name has not been completely forgotten.

6

THE *MUSEUM BRITANNICUM*

"Beware of bees in your bonnet."
Anonymous.

The *Museum Britannicum* is of great significance to the study of the life of Jan Van Rymsdyk, not only because it was the only book published by him, but because in it he reveals his inmost thoughts, and apparently expresses feelings which he had nurtured for many years without expressing them publicly. It was not an official publication, but was published by the author on subscription, and is actually a curious conglomeration of drawings of mainly natural history subjects accompanied by eight-four pages of text. There are thirty plates, some containing more than one figure, and there are numerous footnotes to the text, some extending to more than a page, and swamping the text itself. However, many of them are very revealing, and throw some light on the character of the author.

The editor of the second edition, which was issued by Peter Boyle in 1791, suggests that the original work (1778) had "employed the deceased author Forty-five Years in close study", which would imply that Rymsdyk had been studying natural history since 1733. Since we know little of his activities before 1750, we have no confirmation of this, but he reveals a very early interest in the subject in the text of *Museum Britannicum.*

The British Museum was first opened on 12 January 1759, and the earliest connection between the Museum and Rymsdyk is noted in its Register of Admission to the Reading Room, 1762–1781 (Add. MS. 45869). Under the date 16 July 1772 is recorded: "Mr. Van Rymsdyk to copy Birds, &c. 6 months"; and on 17 February 1774: "Mr. Rymsdyk desire to have their (sic) leave renewed for six months". The preparation of his book, if that is what he had in mind at that time, was taking a long time, and was not published until 1778.

The book was issued with a lengthy, ornate title-page, the type being of varying sizes, and four lines being printed in red. It reads: *Museum Britannicum, being an exhibition of a great variety of antiquities and natural curiosities, belonging to that noble and magnificent cabinet, the British Museum. Illustrated with curious prints, engraved after the original designs, from nature, other objects, and with distinct explanations of each figure, by John and Andrew Van Rymsdyk, pictors* (Plate 16). A quotation and an engraving of the British Museum are followed by the imprint: *London: Printed by J. Moore, for the authors, Charles-Street, St. James's-Square. 1778.* The volume is a folio printed on good paper, a thicker texture being used for the plates. The back of the title-page is blank and faces a dedication by the author (sic) to the Right Hon. and Hon. the Trustees of the British Museum. The dedication continues on the verso, with full titles of their names, including Lord North, the Earl of Dartmouth, Lord Osborn, "and to the remaining subscribers", concluding: "The Authors, J. and A. Van Rymsdyk." Incidentally, this is a rare occasion where Jan Van Rymsdyk's name is given as John.

The preface, "To the Reader" (pp. i–xiii), gives a history of the British Museum, and includes its regulations for use. Rymsdyk begins his vituperations and his critical footnotes in this preface, belabouring the Royal Academy, the lawyers, doctors, social conditions, and virtually every institution and profession mentioned. On engravers he writes (p. viii):

> "I have employed those I thought were men of merit, and able to execute the prints in the manner and taste of the original drawings; they are not engraved with strokes and hatches, as I thought them not natural, that mechanical manner of engraving, or cutting the copper with large broad hatches, grate-like work, I detest. – I encouraged them with sufficient generosity, fixed my own price, and kept nothing secret from them in respect of art, &c. that their performance might give full satisfaction: and on their side they have taken the utmost pains, and every nerve has been stretched to show their art, and good judgement: I venture to say all this in their commendation, and that my drawings were as *intricate* to them *as Nature was to me.* I desired of the engravers** to be very exact in imitating the drawings, for what is all the finest engraving in the world if the drawing is incorrect? Is it not like a body without a soul? or a fine purse without money? – In fine, the drawing is the quintessence, and the engraving with hatches only the mechanical part of the Art." (p. viii).

However, the two stars following the word "engravers" denote the inevitable footnote on the subject:

> "The drawings were engraved by Messrs. Elias Martin, Frederick Martin,

MUSEUM BRITANNICUM,

BEING AN

EXHIBITION

OF A GREAT VARIETY OF

ANTIQUITIES AND NATURAL CURIOSITIES,

BELONGING TO

THAT NOBLE AND MAGNIFICENT CABINET,

THE

BRITISH MUSEUM.

ILLUSTRATED WITH

CURIOUS PRINTS,

Engraved after the ORIGINAL DESIGNS, from NATURE, other OBJECTS;

AND WITH DISTINCT

EXPLANATIONS OF EACH FIGURE,

By JOHN and ANDREW VAN RYMSDYK, PICTORS.

When *Cicero* went to consult the *Oracle* about his future Conduct in Life, he received for Answer,

Follow Nature!

" *No more you learned Fops, your Knowledge boast,*
" *Pretending all to know, by reading most,*
" *True Wit, by Inspiration, we obtain,*
" *Nature, not Art, Apollo's Wreath must gain.*

Mrs. A. BEHN,
in Æsop's Life, 7th Plate.

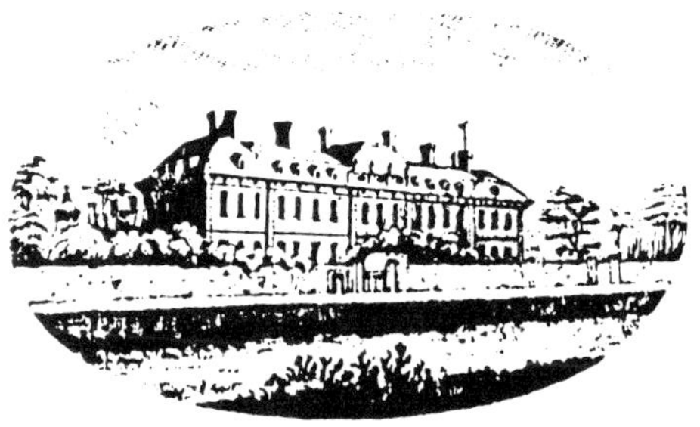

LONDON:

Printed by I. MOORE, for the AUTHORS, CHARLES-STREET,
ST. JAMES'S-SQUARE. 1778.

Plates 16–17 Title-pages of the two editions of *Museum Britannicum* by Jan and Andrew Van Rymsdyk, 1778 and 1791.

> and Charles White, and others. The two last were those who best comprehended the general maxims I made use of in my drawings: and it would have made me still happier if they had been intirely done according to my doctrine; but such is the force of education, that use is a second nature, and there is no hopes (sic) whatsoever for to make them unlearn their old manners. Whatever liquor is thrown into a new vessel, it always will smell of it afterwards: moreover this justifies the old proverb: that, 'An old dog will learn no tricks'. – I had likewise the assistance in the engraving and printing part of this work, of some French frothy snakes. – All the drawings and engravings, are throughout equally finished, whereas most authors, ancient and modern, give only the finest prints in the beginning of their works, the remainder very slight and by indifferent artists."

Rymsdyk follows this by mentioning his son's assistance in the project. Andrew "delineated the title plate from nature, (a North East View of the British Museum)", and eleven other plates, with part of another. Rymsdyk then complains about the cost of the venture:

> "It was my intention to have given a *great-deal* for the money, but the expences of *engraving, letter-press &c.* run very high nowadays; I speak from what I have experienced." (p. ix).

Three pages later he berates "brazen authors, or bookthieves" who do not quote their sources, and "idle thieving Plagiary Drones, and Critick Stinging Wasps." (p. xii).

The index (pp. xiii–xvi) precedes the text and plates. Printed in double columns, it is an index to the text etc., and is not a list of the plates. The thirty plates and eighty-four pages of text terminate with an "Apology of the Author" for any errors.

Although we do not know precisely where Jan Van Rymsdyk was born, this book refers on several pages in general terms to Holland and the Dutch, and he was certainly not of German origin as has been suggested. He quotes Dutch proverbs; for example, in a footnote (p. 60): "The Hollanders have a Proverb, viz. *Considering* is all, said the Maid, and she made but one Bed and laid with her Master."

Betsy Copping Corner (1951) has suggested that Rymsdyk attacked William Hunter in this book under the guise of "Doctor Ibis", and her suggestion is probably well-founded. Hunter had given Rymsdyk scanty recognition for his remarkable drawings in his *Gravid uterus,* and although Rymsdyk made many more drawings for both William and John Hunter, he rather fancied himself as a portrait painter. He had painted or drawn William Smellie in 1753, and several portraits in Bristol during the seventeen-sixties, but possibly he would have liked William Hunter to have used his influence to recommend him to potential clients among the upper classes, and even to sit himself for Rymsdyk. Probably William Hunter was a better judge of Rymsdyk's talents as a medical artist compared with his ability as a portrait painter, and decided on the former. In this capacity he was certainly more useful to William Hunter, and Rymsdyk never forgave him. He wrote:

> "I flatter myself that I have been very useful as a Designer, and Sacrificed my Talents to a good purpose, more so than any Painter in my Profession in this Kingdom; though I look on myself as a Man that has been ill used and Betrayed, the *Author* of my intended *Ruin* is now at my *Mercy,* and I was Advised not to shew him any; but I will rather use *Doctor Ibis*,* as we commonly do a Cur when he barks at the Moon,
>
> *'Now Caps for Men, are thrown to hit,*
> *If it fits you, You may wear it.'*
>
> Neither shall we behave like the Dogs, *who bite on the Stone* without looking *at Him* who threw it, but bear all things with a Manly Patience. On that account, and this the only reason, which I took a dislike to the *Anatomical* Studies, &c. in which I was employed, for I found no relief *from those* as could do me Justice; I submitted, did not resist, and I fell.
>
> *'Tho' Virtue like the Sun, whom Clouds confine,*
> *Or veil'd in Night, may sometimes cease to shine,*
> *Yet when at length its Beames around are hurl'd*
> *It Pleases, and Instructs the duller World.'*
>
> Mrs. A. Behn in *Æsop's life.*
>
> However, I was resolved not to be Idle, I drew and Wrote these Figures and Explanations. . ." (p. 83).

A footnote on Doctor Ibis reads:

> "It is a great comfort to me that he is *Alive,* and will see the above, for I perfectly agree with *Plancus,* who said by way of scoff, 'that none but vain Bugs and Hobgoblins used to fight with the Dead.' Now if this should be answered, (but I believe not) I desire He would take an Example by Me, and write it Himself; for as to employing of other People to write for one, there is something so detestable and cowardly in that; and it is a dishonest mean cunning, in making one self a great Man with other People's Merit. (This is what the Country People call *Reaping without Sowing*). Pray now, as you was (sic) very lucky, and did well

in the World, what Prejudice did I ever do you, why should you discourage me as a Painter; was I not to live too? O if I had a mind to speak how could I expose you, in what we commonly Term a whole length. - But ******** ****** &c. &c. And you have now (I dare say) to your great sorrow and Mortification, lost a useful Subject; Go: and read your Picture in the Fable of the Man and his Goose."

Thus ends the text of the *Museum Britannicum,* but earlier in the book there is a further, possibly indirect reference to William Hunter, again in a footnote (p. 15):

"... as I have seen of a hen, when I made a picture in Crayons of the Progression of the Chicken in a Hen's Egg: which, it is but lately I have been informed the *Best of Women* has in her possession, the most entertaining Picture I ever have done, though it was cunningly kept as a secret from me, in a mean and contemptible manner, that it was intended for our Most Gracious Queen, and this is the reason I could and would not draw any more. – If this is the way that Painters are to be encouraged, *Adieu to all Arts,* and all such professions which have a connection with, and dependency on it; must he not detest the *Art?* will not oppression make a sensible man mad? – The above Picture was done in the best years of my life – who will do a better? I would have done miracles in the art (If the expression may be allowed) had I been properly encouraged. – My Printer is waiting for this. . ."

This reference to the drawings in the possession of the Queen is explained by the fact that the Observatory at Kew was opened in 1769, and was not only used for astronomical observations, but contained a museum. Both George III and Queen Charlotte were interested in the project, which was employed for educational purposes by their children. The Queen was particularly interested in natural history, and various people presented specimens to the museum, including John Hunter, who gave twenty-eight anatomical specimens. In return, the Queen presented him with a small white bull, with which he used to wrestle, until on one occasion he was overpowered, and by good fortune rescued from an awkward predicament. The museum at Kew Observatory was dispersed in 1841, and the anatomical specimens were offered to the Royal College of Surgeons, which housed John Hunter's remarkable collection. Seventy specimens were sent to the College, and included the twenty-eight donated by John Hunter. There was some dispute over the Rymsdyk drawings, as duplicates were to be given to King's College, and William Clift compared the Kew drawings with those already in the Hunterian Museum at the Royal College of Surgeons. He found that the latter contained twenty-five figures and the former twenty-four, but they were judged to be duplicates. However, we have been unable to prove that they went to King's College, or to locate them elsewhere.

It appears probable that Rymsdyk had made the original drawings for John Hunter, and had subsequently copied them. When Rymsdyk discovered them to be in the possession of the Queen, whom William Hunter had attended, he may have assumed that the latter had given them to her, hence his indignation, which appears to have been misdirected. Jessie Dobson (1951) has written the history of the Hunter specimens at Kew Observatory an brought the saga up-to-date. Only five of the specimens received from Kew in 1841 survive, and they have been suitably inscribed and shelved together.

We do not know if Rymsdyk's *Museum Britannicum* was a financial success, and we doubt if it enhanced his reputation as an author or artist. However, it went into a second edition in 1791 (Plate 17). The editor was Peter Boyle, who later edited publications such as *Boyle's Court Guide,* 1792–1808; *The General London Guide, or Tradesman's directory for the year 1794; Boyle's City Guide,* 1797; *Boyle's View of London, and its environs,* (1799); and *The Ladies' Complete Visiting Guide, containing directions for footmen and porters,* (1800?). The title-page of this edition reads: *Museum Britannicum; or a display in thirty-two plates, in antiquities and natural curiosities, in that noble and magnificent cabinet, the British Museum, after the original designs from nature, by John and Andrew Van Rymsdyk, pictors. The second edition, revised and corrected by P. Boyle. Dedicated (by permission) to His Royal Highness the Prince of Wales. (Coat of Arms). London: Printed for the Editor, by J. Moore, No. 134 Drury-Lane. And sold by T. Hookham, Bond-Street, MDCC, XCI.*

A very fulsome dedication, signed by Boyle, is followed by The Advertisement which reads:

> "He has spared no Expence in having the Plates carefully examined, and approved, by the most celebrated Engravers of the Day, notwithstanding the Reduction of Price, from Three Guineas and a half to One Guinea and a half; nor has he been deficient in the painful Task of correcting the Preface, the various Explanations, &c.
>
> Relying, however, on the Indulgence of the liberal and enlightened, the Editor is bold enough to wish this Republication to be accepted as an Earnest of the Work upon the FINE ARTS, now under the Inspection of the First Historical Painter in this, or any other, Kingdom. The Work, alluded to, employed the deceased author Forty-Five years in close Study, and is deemed by those of the Cognoscenti, who have inspected it, one of the most valuable Compositions, ever offered to the Public, and one which has been deeply traced, and clearly investigated, than any heretofore published."

MUSEUM BRITANNICUM;

OR, A DISPLAY

IN THIRTY TWO PLATES,

IN

ANTIQUITIES AND NATURAL CURIOSITIES,

IN

THAT NOBLE AND MAGNIFICENT CABINET,

THE

BRITISH MUSEUM,

AFTER THE ORIGINAL DESIGNS FROM NATURE,

BY JOHN AND ANDREW VAN RYMSDYK, PICTORS.

THE SECOND EDITION, REVISED AND CORRECTED
BY P. BOYLE.

DEDICATED

(*BY PERMISSION*)

TO HIS ROYAL HIGHNESS

THE PRINCE OF WALES.

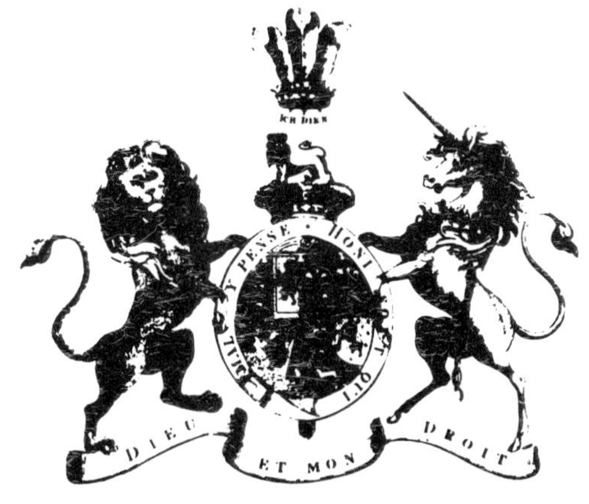

LONDON:
PRINTED FOR THE EDITOR, BY J. MOORE, No. 134, DRURY-LANE.
And Sold by T. HOOKHAM, *Bond-Street*.
M,DCC,XCI.

This is signed by P. Boyle and dated September, which indicates that Jan Van Rymsdyk was dead by then. The lower price would be possible because the original blocks were used, and the editor did not have to pay the original engravers. The plates are also reproduced on inferior paper.

The Preface to the Reader has been slightly curtailed and modified from that in the first edition, and although a few errors have been corrected in the work, others have been introduced. Boyle provides the names and numbers of several items of the late Sir Hans Sloane, and an abstract of Sir Willam Hamilton's collection of antiquities. Five unnumbered pages contain the names of subscribers, including the Prince of Wales and the Duke of York, who head the alphabetical list.

The Wellcome Historical Medical Library contains both editions of the book, but few of the engravings have been improved by being coloured. In fact, Plates IX–X are not the original engravings coloured over, but are specially drawn on different paper, possibly because the originals were too black. These two coloured plates are the most attractive in the collection.

The original drawings for the plates and other illustrations are in the British Museum, having been acquired by purchase as recently as 1948. Those executed by Andrew have been listed in Chapter 7. Sometimes several drawings were engraved on one plate, and occasionally they are signed and dated. Many of the objects on the drawings are numbered, not always consecutively, and the engraved figures are not always arranged to correspond with the drawings. Jan Van Rymsdyk contributed extensive descriptions of the plates. These are not bare annotations such as would be found as captions to museum objects, but indicate a wide range of scholarship on the part of the author. This appears to confirm the suggestion that Jan Van Rymsdyk had been keenly interested in the subject for many years, and it is possible that the opening of the British Museum had prompted him to enlarge upon the knowledge he had acquired, and to publish the book as an unofficial guide to the newly opened Museum. The following list is confined to the illustrations by Jan Van Rymsdyk:

Table I, Figure 1, Taylor-bird's nest from Bengal. Figure 2, Section of a Wasp's nest, given by Dr. John Fothergill.

Table II, Oculus Mundi (Pearls). The original drawing is inscribed: "John Van Rymsdyk Fecit. London, Aug. 31th (sic) – 1772", but on the original drawing the top figure is the drawing by Andrew of the front of the British Museum, which appears on the title-page.

Table III, Incrustated Scull and Sword. Both of these were found in the Tiber in Rome, and are featured on two separate drawings.

Table IV, Ensigns, &c. Figure 1 is possibly a brass ornament such as those found on the bottom of quivers, etc. Figures 2 and 3 are brass ensigns, one of an eagle, the other of a boar, both from Sir William Hamilton's Collection. Figure 4 is a brass spear head from Scotland, and was found at Bannock-Burn. Figures 5–9 are arrow heads, four being of brass, and one of flint.

Table V, Ova, Eggs, features fifteen birds' eggs, and should be compared with Table VI, drawn by Andrew, to show the similarity between the work of the two artists (Plates 18–19).

Table VI, Flagello, bastinado, and Spanish dagger, consists of four figures for which there are two separate original drawings.

Table VII, Spider's Nest, with the Valve. The first two figures are of the nest, Figure 3 shows the silky web, with some of it spun, and Figure 4 is of a piece of garter woven from the silk.

Table XIII, Brick from the Tower of Babel. Figure 1 shows an unburnt brick of about twelve and a half inches square and five inches thick, which was taken from the foundations of the supposed Tower of Babylon. Figure 2, Vas Ægyptium, a canopus with head of Osiris or hawk, in white alabaster with hieroglyphics painted in black. Figure 3, Canopus, the cover a dog's head. Figure 4, Egyptian ring.

Table XV. The Sallad Earthen Vessel, and the Scythian Lamb. Figure 1 features a porous earthen vessel with furrows, which were intended to be covered with the seeds of salad herbs. When the vessel was filled with water the seeds sprouted. Figure 2 is described as a "plant animal called by the Muscovite, Little Lamb." It is actually the root of a fern-like plant. These figures are from two separate drawings.

Table XVII, Tali, Tessera, or Dice. The ten figures represent various types of dice made of lead, bone, brass (2), green jasper, crimson agate, ivory (2), crystal, and dark green agate.

Table XVIII, Amulets, or Charms. Figures 1 and 4 are of Druid amulets in enamelled glass, and were presented to the Museum by Jacob Bell, a Quaker. Figures 2 and 3 are captioned "Ithyphalliques", trinkets to be worn on watches and on the hair. Figure 5 is a round crystal ball amulet.

Table XX, Figure 2 is a glass tumbler with the bottom portion encrusted with a chalk-like substance.

Table XXI, Lachrymatories, or Tear-Vials, to contain the tears of weeping friends, and which were buried with the dead. Figures 1 and 2 are glass, and 3 is of red terra cotta.

Table XXIII, Graptolithi, Figured Slates, and an Agat, with the Eclipse of the Sun. Figure 1 depicts a "Derby or Florentine Stone, on which by the hand of Nature is depicted a beautiful landscape". Figure 2, "The

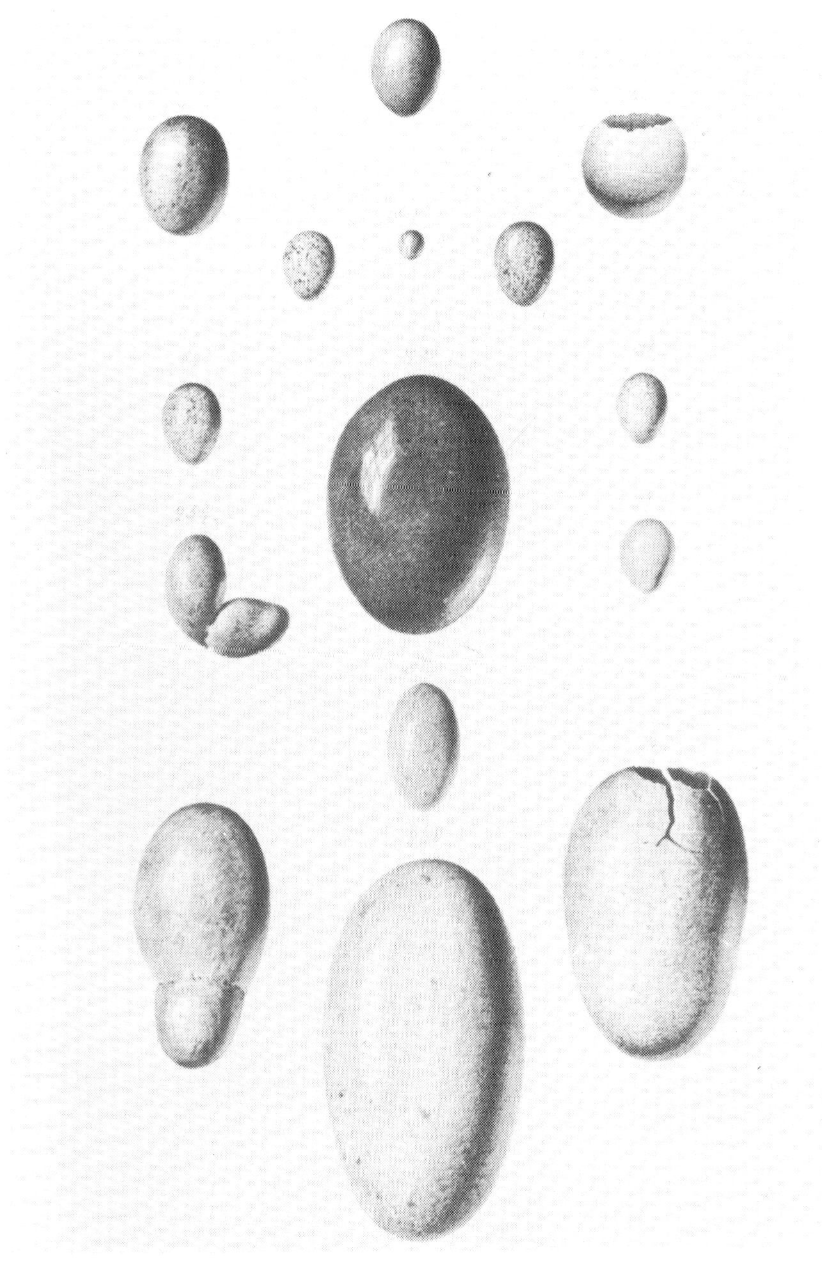

Plates 18–19 Original drawings for Plates V and VI of *Museum Britannicum.* Plate V is by Jan, and Plate VI is by Andrew Van Rymsdyk (British Museum).

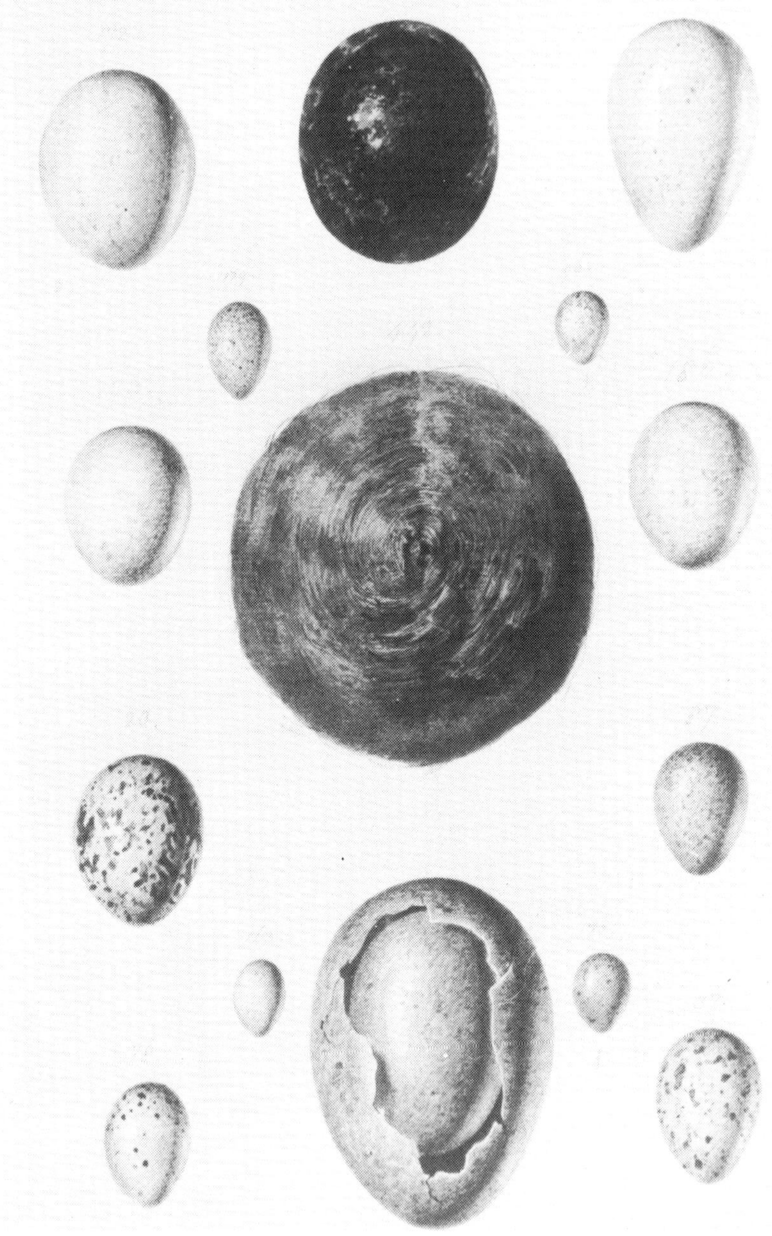

India Agat, a pendant, set in form of a heart, here Nature again has drawn on it a true representation of an eclipse of the sun, and the moon"; on the bottom hangs an onyx drop.

Table XXV, Greek and Roman Tesserae, or Tickets. Figure 1 depicts a hand in relief, with thumb and first finger raised, and is in ivory. Figure 2 depicts a bone cut in the form of a ram's head. Figure 3 is an ivory theatre ticket set in a silver frame. Figure 4 is an ivory ticket and Figure 5 is a crystal ticket. Figures 6 and 7 are tickets of the same size, inscribed with a name, possibly that of a play.

Table XXVI. A roman Patera, & a large golden one ditto. Figure 1 shows a shallow red Roman patera, pocullum, or little cup, which was found at Black Stakes, near Chatham. Figure 2 is a large gold patera dedicated to Baccus, found at Gergenti, Sicily, and was from Sir William Hamilton's Collection.

Table XXVII, Nautilus Papyraceus, or paper nautilus. Figure 1, The fish, a cast from nature in wax, placed in the natural shell. Figure 2, Purpera, a shell, and figure 3, also a shell, Wendel or Wentel Trap, "so named by Hollanders", but in this country called "the Royal Staircase". Figure 4, Echini Marini, the sea hedgehog, or urchin. The centre, unnumbered, figure on the engraved plate (top figure in the original drawing) is captioned "real sails and legs from a dried and dissected Nautilus", and was probably drawn by Andrew.

Table XXVIII, Governor Pitt's Brilliant Diamond, &c, features a model of the uncut stone (Figure 1), and in Figures 2 and 3 drawings from casts in metal of the first and second cutting, while Figure 4 is a model of Pitt's diamond. Figure 5 is a model of the Duke of Tuscany's diamond, a diagram of which is shown in Figure 7. Figures 6 and 8 are diagrams of the diamonds respectively of the King of France and the Empress of Russia. Figure 9 is a separate original drawing, and is of a rough Egyptian pebble broken obliquely in half.

Table XXIX, Antiquitates Ægyptiacae, Sistrum, &c. Figure 1 is the sistrum, an ancient musical instrument or rattle made of copper. Figures 2 and 3 are figurines of Osiris and Isis, and the originals are on a sheet of paper containing a ram's head in a circle, described on page 79 as "Mendes, or Pan, a vignet", but reproduced at the bottom of page 44; and a pin drawn by Andrew. In the second edition the ram's head is printed on page X at the end of the Preface, with an added crest and the motto "Ich Dien".

Table XXX, Aves, Birds. Figures 1 to 3 are of humming birds from America, with one bird on a nest, and two separate eggs. Figure 4,

Paradisca Regia, or the Kings Bird of Paradise.

A separate drawing is reproduced on page 78 of the text, and is described as, "An Ibis, preserved by the Egyptians in an earthen red cylindrical pott, or urn, sealed up with a white cement. . . . Given to Sir H. Sloane by my Lord Sandwich, who brought it from the Pyramids of Egypt."

When describing the various specimens Rymsdyk frequently quotes references to authorities, indicating that he had read widely in French, German and Latin, in addition to his native Dutch and adopted English. However, one footnote (p. 82) does not give a source for the information, and gives rise to an interesting speculation. When describing humming birds he provides information on blossoms:

> ". . . after a great drought in Jamaica, the Blossoms being shut covered with dust. . .; it had not rained for some time, a gentle shower came at last in the evening. . .; There was a Tree in my Garden full of Blossoms, facing my Back Parlour, which was covered, and hovered over immediately with a multitude of half starved different species of Humming Birds, as many as there were Blossoms, sucking their Food; (*etc.*).

This suggests that Jan Van Rymsdyk might himself have visited Jamaica, and this might have been while he was living in Bristol, which had a regular trade with the West Indies. This is the only reference to a possible trip outside England after he settled there.

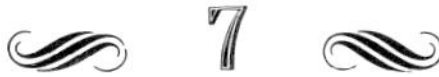

ANDREW VAN RYMSDYK (1753 or 1754-1786)

"The more we study, we the more discover our ignorance".
Shelley.

We know as little of the life of his son as of Jan Van Rymsdyk himself. In fact, it was only recently that we were able to deduce the approximate date of his birth. Knowing that he had received awards from the Royal Society of Arts, we investigated their records and discovered vital clues in Robert Dossie's *Memoirs* (1782) and in the Society's "Minutes of Committees, 1766–7".

The Society of Arts was founded in 1754 and played an important part in the promotion of the arts and of agriculture. It awarded premiums to artists and inventors, and the history of its extensive activities have been recorded by Hudson and Luckhurst (1954) and Allan (1974). Dossie (1782) gives "A list of premiums, bounties and rewards, bestowed on various subjects in drawing, etching, engraving, painting and modelling, encouraged by the Society for the Improvement of Arts, &c. . . . from the time of the Institution, to the year 1776, in the class of polite arts" (p. 404), and this proved a useful source of information, as indicated by the following extracts:

> "1765. Andr. van Rymsdyk, aged 11 years, son of Mr. John Van Rymsdyk, Painter of History and other Subjects, Wych-str. Dru. Lane, *Copy of the* Tribute-money, after P. P. Rubens, of 20Gs. Prem. 8 Guineas".

This is followed by three other names, with premiums of five, four and three guineas respectively, suggesting that of a total of twenty guineas, Andrew received the highest premium. In the following year he received half of the total, viz.:

> "Andries van Rymsdyk, aged 12. Transfiguration, after Raphael, 10 Guineas", followed by two other names with sums of six and four guineas respectively.

These entries suggest that Andrew was at this time known as Andries or

Andreas, but more significantly they give his age in each of these years. By deduction we can assume that he was born in either 1753 or 1754, depending upon the month of his birth and the actual dates of the awards. His name also appears in the awards for 1767:

"Andr. van Rymsdyk, a Drawing, *Conversion of St. Paul, after Rubens,* Bounty, a Silver Pallet gilt", the only name appearing under this Class, but under the heading Mezzotintos we find:

"Andries van Rymsdyk, a dead Christ, after Sir A. van Dyck, a well executed piece, dedicated, by permission, to the Society, out of gratitude and respect, by the young Artist". Three other names follow this, with awards of twelve, eight and five guineas.

The Minutes of Committees, 1766–7, give further information on the award of the Bounty to Andrew:

> "January 16th. Opened the Papers containing the Names of the Candidates who have gained Premiums. . . . Drawing of Human Figure Class 96. Silver Pallet gilt appeared to be done by Andrew Van Rymsdyk at Mr. Butler's in Broad Street Carnaby Market. February 5th. Class 96. Andrew Van Rymsdyk at Mr. Butler's in Broad Street Carnaby Market, to whom Silver Gilt Pallet was given as a Bounty, attended and received his Bounty."

Andrew Van Rymsdyk exhibited at the Society of Artists of Great Britain, which had been founded in 1760, and after it had been founded in 1769, at the Royal Academy of Arts. His exhibits are listed by Graves (1906 and 1907); and the addresses given are possibly where he was living at the time:

1769. Society of Artists. *Charles Street, St. James's*
    148. A portrait.
    149. A piece of still life. (Graves (1907, p. 221))
1775. Royal Academy of Arts. (Under heading "RYMSDYK, A.V. . . . Painter 84 East Queen Anne Street, Cavendish Square"
    269. La Patesser or Patty-man. *Vid.* Yorrick's Sentimental Journey, p. 46.
    270. Rennes, or the sword. *Vid.* Yorrick's Sentimental Journey, p. 54.
    271. Portrait of a lady. (Graves (1906, p. 54).
1776. Society of Artists. *89 East Queen Anne Street, Cavendish Square.*
    82. Hotspur having defeated Douglas at Holmden Hill. See Shakespear's Henry IV, Act II, Scene IV.
    83. The Battle of Agincourt, representing the Earl of Exeter supporting Edward, Duke of York who is expiring near the body

of his Deceased Friend, Lord Suffolk. See Shakespear's Henry V, Act IV.

84. Portrait, three quarters.

260. Portrait of a lady; in chalk.

261. Ditto.

345. Portrait of a Lady, small whole length.

346. A Nymph bathing. (Graves (1907, p. 221))

1778. Royal Academy of Arts. (Under heading "RYMSDYK, -Junr., Enamel Painter at Mr. Frewin's, Porter Street, Soho. (Graves (1906, p. 398))

168. A lady in a fancy dress; enamel

169. Head of King Lear; do.

At the end of 1758 and in 1759 Jan Van Rymsdyk was living in Bristol, and he was probably still there in 1762 and 1764 when he painted portraits of Bristol personalities. Andrew may have been with him at this period, but Jan was also making numerous drawings for William Hunter in 1764, and must have been in London when depicting the complicated dissections. The British Museum was opened to the public on 12 January 1759, and a few years later Jan Van Rymsdyk must have decided to draw some of the exhibits with a view to publishing *Museum Britannicum* (see Chapter 6). In July 1772 he was given permission "to copy Birds, &c." for six months, and this was renewed for a similar period in February 1774. The permit probably also covered his son Andrew, and this period would partly account for the gap in Andrew's exhibiting. Jan Van Rymsdyk detailed the contributions of his son to the *Museum Britannicum,* mentioning verse quotations in addition to his drawings for the plates. The original drawings are in the British Museum, having been purchased in 1948, and they have been compared with the engravings. Few of the drawings are signed or dated, none by Andrew, and it is impossible to distinguish between the technique of father and son. This is specially notable in Plates V and VI, both of birds' eggs, the first by Jan and the second by Andrew (Plates 12–13).

Some of the drawings contain several figures on a page, and occasionally more than one single-page drawing was engraved as a multiple figure on a plate. In the original drawings, many of the individual figures are numbered, but the numbering has no obvious significance. Andrew was the artist responsible for the drawings for the following plates, which are designated tables in the book; and he also drew the vignette of the Museum which appears on the title-page of the first edition. The vignette appears at the top of the drawings for Table II, and the original sheet is signed and dated "John Van

Rymsdyk Fecit. London Aug. 31th (sic) – 1772". It is possible that Andrew's drawing for the title page was added later in the first blank space on the drawing which would appear near the front of the book.

Table VI, Ova, eggs, consists of fifteen figures, all but one being of birds' eggs. Figure 7, in the centre of the Table, is of a hair ball in an ox's stomach, from Jamaica.

Table VII, Annuli, rings, contains thirteen figures depicting rings made from iron, agate, brass, gold, silver and jasper.

Table IX, Penknife with a gold point, and copper horse-shoe. In Figure 1 the knife has an agate handle, and the gold was supposed to have been made by transmutation. Figure 2 represents a horse-shoe to have been taken out of water from copper-mines in Hungary.

Table X, Stylus and Roman Fibulae, consists of eight figures, but there is no drawing of Figure 1, and Figure 2 is with a group of three others on a separate sheet. Two of these are on Table XXIX, (Figures 2 and 3), and the third appears as a separate vignette on the bottom of page 44 of the text. This represents a ram's head in a circle, and the caption (on page 79) described it as "Mendes, or Pan". In the second edition of the *Museum Britannicum* this vignette is on page X at the end of the Preface, with an added crest with the motto "Ich Dien"! It is possible that all these were drawn by Andrew, and also another small illustration in the text (page 78), which is described as "An Ibis, preserved by the Egyptians in an earthen red cylindrical pott, or urn, sealed up with a white cement". It was given to Sir Hans Sloane by Lord Sandwich, "who brought it from the Pyramids of Egypt."

Table XI, *Pinna Marina,* a shell. This is illustrated in Figure 1, and Figure 2 illustrates "a pair of men's gloves made from the beard of the *Pinna marina,* from Andalusia in Spain."

Table XIV, Amulets, or charms. Figure 1 is a *"purse like Bullae"*, of gold, Figure 2 is an Egyptian amulet, a scarab, and Figure 3 shows the back of this inscribed with hieroglyphics, which were not then understood. This is carved on "a black stone, like our slate."

Table XVI, *Nidus Gelatinus,* or Soup-Nest. Figure 1 shows the front of a swallow's nest from Cambodia, and Figure 2 a spary bird's nest with eggs and twigs encrusted with "a fine sparkling spar."

Table XIX, Calculi, Stones. Figure 1 shows calculus surrounding a silver bodkin; Figure 2, a bezoar nut from "East India"; Figures 3 and 4, Monkey's bezoars; Figure 5, a calculus, "the nucleus a plumb-stone"; and Figure 6, a "round serpent-stone."

Table XX, A Coral Hand. Figure 1 illustrates a curious coral, "modled by nature in the form of a hand or glove, with round perforations." Figure 2 is a glass tumbler, "under part incrusted with a limey or stoney subtance."

Table XXII, Lamps, and the Asbestos. Figure 1 depicts a "sepulchral lamp of gray earth or clay", with a bear in relief, and Figure 2 shows a lamp with three nozzles. Figure 3 illustrates "the real fossile Asbestos", and Figure 4 shows a purse made of asbestos.

Table XXIV. Human Horn, and the Crotalum. Figure 1 shows one of the horns of "Mrs. French of Tenterden", who had a horny substance growing from the back of her head. Figure 2 is of a crotalum, a kind of cymbal, with eight round plates of bronze or brass.

Table XXVII, *Nautilus Papyraceus,* or paper nautilus. Andrew was responsible for only part of this plate, which contains five figures, one of which (that in the centre) is unnumbered. From its position on the original drawing, and from comparison with the others, it would appear that this was probably by Andrew. It is of the "real sails and legs from a dried and dissected Nautilus."

Andrew appears to have decided to concentrate on painting miniatures, and was probably responsible for executing many of which no records exist. Some probably remain unrecognised in private hands, for many were unsigned, and the names of the subjects are not known. He appears to have visited various resorts at intervals, advertising his services and remaining in the locality while work was available, but Bath was apparently his main base from 1781 to 1786.

Bryan Little (1980) has provided an interesting insight into the history of Bath, which was established as England's premier watering place long before the eighteenth century. It was patronised by royalty, bishops, politicians, professional men and gentry, and in 1702 and 1703 Queen Anne stayed there. Shortly afterwards, Richard Nash, later to become known as Beau Nash, went to Bath and soon dominated by his personality the theatre, gambling and all other social activities in the spa. Members of the aristocracy from all over the country flocked there, and Bath became the fashionable centre for holidays long before visits to the seaside became the vogue. Buildings were renovated, lodgings were improved, and the town rapidly grew to accommodate the increasing population. Its proximity to Bristol ensured the supply of building materials, provisions for the visitors, and the port was within easy reach for the merchants. The Baths themselves were renovated, the Circus, the Crescent, and many other areas were developed, including the erection of several imposing public buildings. Merchants, shopkeepers, craftsmen, actors and artists were attracted to supply the needs of the community, and it was probably the possibility of finding customers among the visitors that prompted Andrew Van Rymsdyk to settle in Bath as a miniature-portrait painter.

The issue of *Bath Chronicle* for 22 February 1781 printed the notice: "Mr. Rymsdyk, miniature painter and M.R.A. at Mrs. Smith, Ladymead". Although

Andrew had exhibited at the Royal Academy, he was not elected to the Membership, and should not have described himself as M.R.A. A miniature of an unknown lady, signed and dated, "Drawn by Andrew Rymsdyk, 1781", was in the collection of Miss D. M. Kleinfeldt", (Foskett, 1972, Plate 313) and the same source reproduces another "Unknown lady", (Plate 314). These are both oval-shaped, 5¼ and 4⅞ inches respectively. Also in 1781, Andrew visited Norwich, and *The Norfolk Chronicle* for 13 October recorded: "Mr. Rymsdyk, miniature painter, Member of the Royal Academy, London, has arrived in Norwich." Two years later he went to Chester, and *Adam's Weekly Courant* for 22 July 1783 carried the advertisement: "Van Rymsdyk, miniature painter and Member of the Royal Academy, London, visits Chester. He draws likenesses &c, 1 guinea each." He was back in Bath later the same year, and on 16 October 1783 the *Bath Chronicle* printed the notice: "Portraits in a new style. Andrew Rymsdyk painter in miniature most respectfully acquaints that he draws accurate likenesses of all ages. Price 1½ guineas frame and glass included. Specimens of his drawings may be seen at his house at Mr. Dawson's St. James' Street". The same newspaper carried similar notices on 28 October, and 2 and 18 November 1784, but he was then living at No. 6, King Street, and he mentioned also, "specimens of his drawings to be seen everyday at the Pump Room and at his house". An oval water-colour (6¼ x 2¾ inches), signed: "Painted by Andrew Rymsdyk, 1784", from the Bath Literary Club Collection, 1929, is listed in the Victoria Art Gallery Catalogue of the Permanent Collection as: "Mrs. Richard Tickell and her daughter Elizabeth Ann, born *April 1781,* died in London at Bedford Square, 1860. (Child, (aged 3) on table. Curtain and pillar in background.)"

In 1963 Mary, Countess of Pembroke purchased in Lewes a charming water-colour (13 x 15 inches) signed and dated "Andrew Rymsdyk 1786." This shows two children and two dogs in a pleasant setting with a church and mansion in the background. The Countess wrote to *Country Life* (18 April 1963) requesting information on the identity of the children and their setting, and her watercolour was reproduced with her letter. In reply she received two letters, one from Alban Bower of Matlock, who suggested that "the park illustrated appears to be Alfreton Park, Derbyshire; . . . which was the seat of the Moorwood family". He further stated that the picture was sold at Alfreton Hall on December 1960, and that several other small water-colours by Andrew Rymsdyk were sold at the same time (Alban Bower, A.L.S., 21 April 1963). Mr. Bower has since died, but his widow, Mrs. Janet M. Bower, informs me (Janet M. Bower, A.L.S., 12 January 1980) that they acquired a water-colour by Andrew at that sale, a small oval about 5 by 4 inches. This is a portrait of Henry Case Morewood, Rector of Ladbrook, Warwickshire, second husband of Ellen

Case Morewood, widow of George Morewood of Alfreton Hall, Derbyshire. A typed slip of paper attached to the back of the water-colour states: "Painted by Andrew Rymsdyk, being a miniature copy of a portion of the portrait in oils by Wright of Derby (the latter signed and dated I.W.P. 1782). N.B. Henry Case inherited the Alfreton Hall Estates on marrying and took the name and arms of Morewood in 1793, and died 1825."

The second letter to the Countess of Pembroke was from the late Mary Aubrey Coker of Mayfield, Sussex (A.L.S. dated 30 June 1963), who stated that she had four water-colour portraits of her Aubrey ancestors painted by Andrew Rymsdyk; also a miniature of Mary Aubrey identical to the water-colour. The miniature, Miss Coker gave to her niece, but the watercolours, of three men and one lady, are now in the possession of Ruth G. Gilmour, also of Mayfield. They are in oval gilt frames (7 x 8½ inches), the inner portraits being 3⅝ x 5½ inches.

The Victoria and Albert Museum has two oval, framed miniatures by Andrew Van Rymsdyk (Nos. 66788 and 67212), one of a man, and the other of an elderly lady. The National Gallery of Ireland, Dublin, contains two others: "Portrait of a child (Earl of Athlone)", (No. 14,547), and "Portrait of a lady (possibly Mrs. Siddons)", (No. 14,548). The former is signed and dated 1783, the latter 1785. The two miniatures went to the Gallery as a long-term loan.

The water-colour owned by the Countess of Pembroke and dated 1786 was probably painted on his last expedition from the city in which he made his home, for on 24 August of that year the *Bath Chronicle* noted: "Mr. Rymsdyk arrives at Bath. Portraits drawn £2.2.0. each". Less than three months later the same newspaper for 16 November recorded his death: "On Monday died at his lodgings in this city Mr. Andrew Rymsdyk, a portrait painter of great merit." We have not been able to trace his burial place, but his father was still alive, and was probably living in London. Andrew was only about thirty-three years old, and before reaching his teens had shown great promise as an artist, but later concentrated on miniatures. Edward Edwards, who probably knew both father and son from having worked on the same specimen as Jan in 1764, wrote of Andrew, ". . . his abilities as an artist were not very powerful" (Edwards, 1808, p. 58). Despite this, Andrew's miniatures are very attractive, and it is probable that if more of his work could be traced, his talent would be more fully appreciated.

8

RYMSDYK'S DRAWINGS FOR THOMAS DENMAN (1733–1815), AND OTHERS

"There is so much truth and elegance in the drawings executed by Mr. Rymsdyk they may be considered as patterns for all future artists."
Thomas Denman.

In his *Museum Britannicum,* Rymsdyk had announced that he would not undertake drawing further medical subjects, and after the publication of that book his activities appeared to have been curtailed. He seemed to have disappeared from the London scene, and at one time it was thought that he had retired either to Bath or Bristol, and probably died there. However, by chance some drawings by him were noticed in publications by Thomas Denman (1733–1815), who had succeeded William Hunter as the leading London obstetrician. Denman, despite his status during his lifetime, and the influence of his work as recorded by his contemporaries and successors, has been badly neglected by most modern historians of obstetrics. There is no biographical study of him, and he is chiefly remembered as the father of a Lord Chief Justice of England, and of the respective wives of Sir Richard Croft and Matthew Baillie. However, in 1779 Denman wrote a memoir "for his descendants, and perhaps relations", which was later continued, possibly by Matthew Baillie, and published in Denman's *Introduction to the practice of midwifery,* sixth edition, London, 1824. This is the main source of information on the career of a remarkable man who made significant contributions to his profession. It was drawn upon by Herbert R. Spencer (1927) when writing about Denman in his *History of British midwifery from 1650–1800* (pp. 128–142).

Thomas Denman was born at Bakewell, Derbyshire, on 27 June 1733, the third child and second son of John and Elizabeth Denman, who later produced five more children, including two sets of twins. Three died in infancy, but John Denman, who was an apothecary, found difficulty in providing for the family, and took to drink and "company". He died aged fifty-eight of dropsy, when his eldest son Joseph was almost twenty-one, and had spent two years studying in London. This son succeeded his father in the business at Bakewell, but it was not very flourishing, and Thomas assisted him for two years. In 1754 Thomas went to London with a small bequest from his grandfather and twenty-five pounds as his share of his father's assets. This money was intended for him to attend St. George's Hospital, but in six months he had spent the lot. He applied to the Navy Board for an order to be examined at Surgeon's Hall, and he passed as surgeon to a ship of sixth rate on 3 April 1755. Denman sailed to Gibraltar, Minorca and Altea, but had two bouts of "hospital fever". Returning to England at the end of 1756, he came to London and met the Dowager Duchess of Devonshire, to whose family at Chatsworth his father had been apothecary for several years. Through her influence he was appointed Surgeon to the *Weazle* and then to the *Centaur*. He visited Guinea, Teneriffe, the West Indies and the Mediterranean on some of his voyages, and was at the sieges of Belle Isle and Havana. Altogether he spent nine years in the Navy, gaining extensive experience as a ship's surgeon, receiving prize money and pay, which he rapidly spent when ashore. Eventually the Fleet returned to Plymouth, and Denman wrote: "I was set at Liberty in the year 1763". He attended lectures on anatomy and midwifery and then settled in Winchester which, he later wrote, contained "more medical men than could live", and he soon left, "having thrown away since my arrival in England nearly two hundred pounds."

Once more Denman came to London, and attended dissections and lectures on anatomy before acquiring an M.D. from Aberdeen. He started to practise, but made little headway and decided to rejoin the Navy, but he was unable to obtain a warrant. He published *Essays on the puerperal fever, and on puerperal convulsions,* London, 1768, and shortly afterwards, *A letter on the construction and use of vapour baths,* 1768. He applied for the post as surgeon on one of the King's yachts, and was appointed to the *William and Mary* at a salary of seventy pounds per annum. This was almost a sinecure and in 1777, when the yacht was ordered upon service, he resigned as "the attendance would have been incompatible with my business in London". Denman took a small house in Oxenden Street. A teacher of midwifery, Dr. Cooper, "of no great reputation", died, and Osborn, who attended St. George's Hospital with Denman, agreed to give lectures on the subject with him. The lectures flourished, and Thomas Denman and Henry Krohn (died 1816) were jointly elected to succeed Cooper as man-wife to Middlesex Hospital.

In his thirty-seventh year Thomas Denman married Elizabeth Brodie, who brought two leasehold houses in Vine Street, Piccadilly, as a dowry. Within a year she also produced twin daughters; Margaret, who in 1789 married

Richard Croft, later knighted; and Sophia, who became the wife of Matthew Baillie in 1791. In 1772 Denman moved to a larger house in Queen Street, Golden Square. His business "was chiefly among the lower class of people", but he soon purchased "a chariot", and had a coachman in handsome livery, with a servant behind. In 1779 his son Thomas was born, described by Denman as an "unexpected blessing". Eventually he was to become Lord Chief Justice of England.

The death of William Hunter in 1783, "raised him into the highest practice, and placed him at the head of his branch of the profession." He moved to Old Burlington Street, and in 1783 attended the Duchess of Devonshire in her confinement. Denman gave up lecturing, and when his practice grew he gradually introduced his son-in-law, Richard Croft, and eventually left him with the business. Thomas Denman died in 1815 aged eighty-two, deeply respected, following a distinguished career which had commenced in a most unprepossessing manner. He had written several important publications, including *Aphorisms on the application and use of the forceps and vectis in preternatural labours, or labours attended with hemorrhage or convulsions,* 1783; *An essay on uterine hemorrhages,* 1786; *An essay on preternatural labours,* 1786; *An essay on natural labours,* 1786; *An introduction to the practice of midwifery,* 2 vols., 1788, which went into numerous editions and translations, and was probably his most important work; *Observations on rupture of the uterus, on the snuffles in infants, and on mania lactea,* 1810; and *Observations on the cure of cancers,* 1810. But from our viewpoint Denman's most important publication was *A collection of engravings, tending to illustrate the generation and parturition of animals, and of the human species,* which was issued as a folio in 1787. In his preface (p. 2) Denman states:

> "Some years ago, without any view to this publication, I began to have drawings taken of such subjects as occurred to me relative to utero-gestation or parturition in the human species, or in animals, natural, preternatural, or morbid; whenever they appeared likely to give a more comprehensive view of the science of Midwifery, or to improve the art; to elucidate such things as were obscurely known; or, to exhibit others which could be more clearly understood by this mode of representation. My collection is not large, but they are all taken from nature; and there is so much truth and elegance in the drawings executed by Mr. Rymsdyk they may be considered as patterns for all future artists. Some of these being engraved, I am unwilling that they should be lost, and therefore publish this first number as a specimen of the work."

Denman further stated that if he was unable to continue the work, it would be conducted by John Clark, teacher of midwifery in Queen-Street.

The *Collection* consists of nine unnumbered plates, the captions facing the plates being in both English and French. Six of them were engraved from original drawings by Rymsdyk, and all bear dates of publication which range from 22 December 1783 (3 plates, one by Rymsdyk) to 23 February 1787 (5 plates, four by Rymsdyk), one other being dated as drawn by Rymsdyk in 1784, and published on 1 November 1786. This is of the human uterus at term (Plate 20), a subject Rymsdyk had earlier depicted for William Hunter in 1750, William Smellie in 1751, and C. N. Jenty in 1757 (Thornton and Want, 1979). The other subjects drawn by Rymsdyk were the funis of a nut, etc.; the internal parts of a frog; a section of a hen; the uterus of a cow; and three human abortions. All the illustrations from Denman's *Collection* were included in the third, 1801, edition of his *Introduction to the practice of midwifery,* together with eight other plates, one of which was drawn by Rymsdyk. They also appeared in later editions of the *Introduction,* and were generally grouped together either following the index or between the list of contents and the actual text. The plates were also issued separately in *Engravings, representing the generation of some animals; some circumstances attending parturition in the human species; and a few of the diseases to which the sex is liable,* a quarto volume published in 1815. In the preface to this Denman wrote:

> "When I first entertained the design of having drawings taken, and plates engraved, it was my intention to make such a collection as would have enabled me to have given specimens of the generation of all the animals I could procure, or favourable accidents might afford; together with representations of the chief circumstances which accompany or follow human parturition, and the diseases to which the female sex is peculiarly liable. But too many avocations have intervened, and these have obliged me to suspend my intention, or rather to give it up in despair; but should I ever resume the pursuit, it would be conducted on the same plan.
>
> Those plates which were executed, were, I believe, well done, and they were placed in the quarto edition of the Introduction to the Practice of Midwifery. But the present Publishers, persuaded that they would be more acceptable if they were edited in a distinct publication, I can make no objection to their proposal, and I hope they may be of some use to Students, and answer their expectations."

In this edition the plates do not bear the date of publication, but the imprint on most of them is "London. Published by E. Cox & Son, St. Thomas's Street, Borough." The plates are not numbered, but the captions on a separate page are. Numbers I–III are the same as in the 1787 edition; IV–IX are as in the *Introduction,* 1801; X is lettered and dated as in the 1787 edition (8), and the 1801 volume (10); XI and XII as in the 1801 publication; XIII as that of 1801,

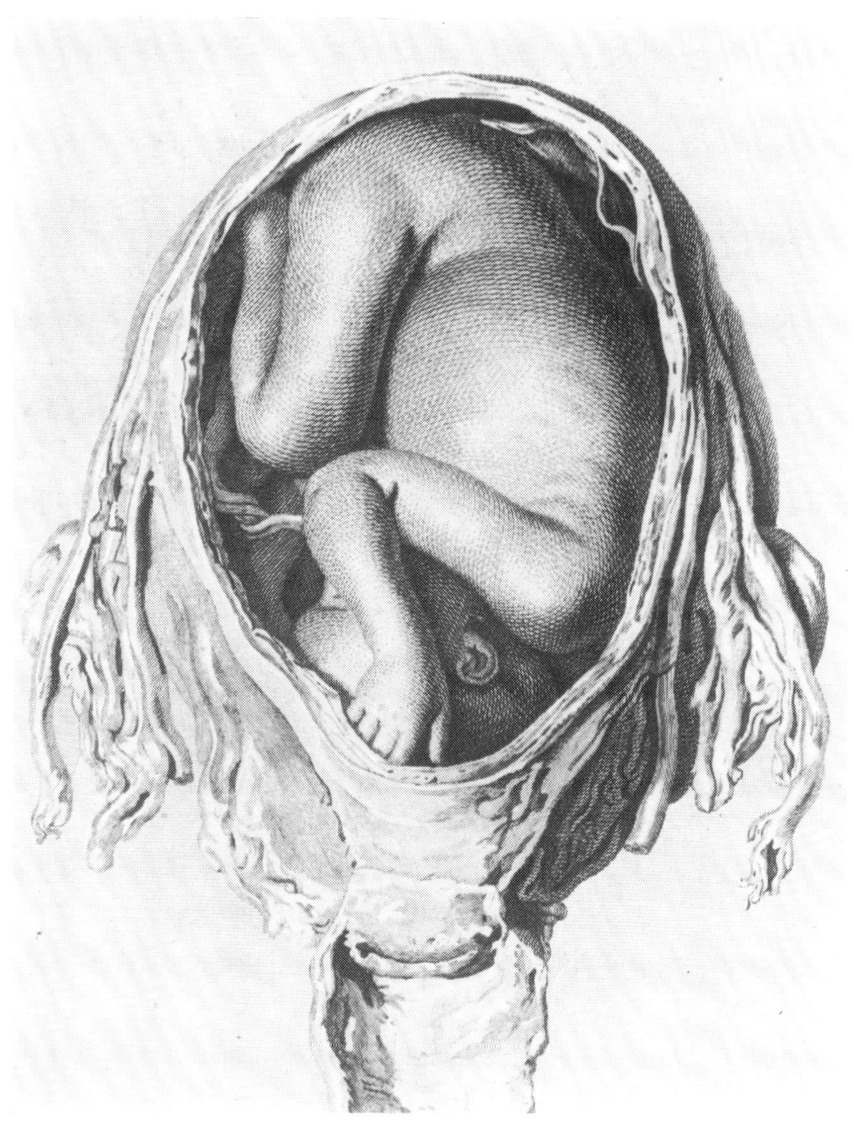

Plate 20 Engraved version of Jan Van Rymsdyk's drawing of the gravid uterus at term, from Thomas Denman's *Collection of engravings,* 1787.

but with the Cox imprint included; XIV–XV the same as 1801; XVII has no lettering whatsoever at the foot of the plate; while XVI is lettered exactly as in the 1801 book, even "Publ. by T. Denman M.D. 2 Feby. 1801."

Plate IV, of "Uterus, with bladder of an ewe", is most important from our view-point because it was drawn by "J. V. Rymsdyk" and the date of publication is given as 23 February 1789, twelve years before its first appearance in Denman's *Introduction* (1801) and two years after his *Collection of engravings* was published in 1787. This suggests that it was probably drawn in 1788, since all the additional plates are dated between 1788 and 1801. This is the latest reference to Jan Van Rymsdyk we have traced, and he probably died in either 1788 or 1789.

Jan Van Rymsdyk made drawings for other people, and a few of these have been traced. The Department of Prints and Drawings at the British Museum houses one with the handwritten inscription "John Van Rymsdyk after Jacob Jordaens; but not a servile imitation. London 1783", and another of the head of an ox, buffalo or moose, as it is variously described. The British Museum (Natural History) have suggested that it might be either the African Buffalo (*Syncerus caffer*), or the Asiatic Buffalo (*Bubalus bubalus*). It is signed and dated "J. V. Rymsdyk, F. 1773", and originally came from the Banks Collection.

He also made the original drawings for the plates in George Macaulay's "An account of a child whose abdominal viscera were chiefly found in the cavity of the thorax" (*Medical Observations and Inquiries,* 1, 1757, pp. 25–35). The originals are dated and signed by Rymsdyk, 5 December 1754; Plate II has an extra figure added in the engraving, and Plate III omits the head and limbs. David Bayford (1739–1790) wrote a paper published as "An account of two aneurysms in the aorta, described by Mr. Bayford and communicated by Dr. William Hunter. Read July 5, 1762" (*Medical Observations and Inquiries,* 3, 1767, pp. 14–27). Rymsdyk made the original drawings for both plates, Plate 1 containing five figures and Plate 2 featuring three figures. Little is known about David Bayford who first described dysphagia lusoria, but N. Asherson (1979), has provided some information on his life and work. Rymsdyk also provided the two figures for the plate illustrating M. Garthshore's "Case of fatal ileus." (*Medical Observations and Inquiries,* 4, 1771, pp. 223–230; plate at end of volume).

It is possible that both Jan and Andrew Van Rymsdyk left many other drawings with their personal effects when they died. Andrew died before his father, who probably inherited Andrew's property, but we do not know where or precisely when Jan died, and no trace of his effects has been found. Both had been experienced artists, and advertised the fact that examples of their work were available to be seen by potential customers, yet nothing remains in public collections to suggest that it was in the possession of the artists at their deaths. No descendants have been recorded, and it is doubtful if there were any, since there is no record of Andrew being married, and as far as we know, he was Jan's only son. The only surviving original material is that commissioned by the Hunters, Smellie, Jenty, the drawings for the *Museum Britannicum,* a few specimens of their work acquired by museums and art galleries, and others still in private hands, as recorded elsewhere.

RYMSDYK'S INFLUENCE ON MEDICAL BOOK ILLUSTRATION

"Dead he is not, but departed, – for the artist never dies."
Longfellow.

The origin of the depiction of medical subjects extends into antiquity, when cave drawings, statuettes fashioned in bone and stone, and stone carvings depicted human subjects. Some of these showed anatomical distortions and abnormalities, which may have been the fault of the artist, or equally well may have been malformations, possibly accenuated by caricature. Injuries can occasionally be identified by the fact that the weapon is depicted *in situ,* and warts, tumours, shortened limbs, and other obvious anatomical defects are readily recognised. William Anderson (1885) published a lengthy lecture on art in its relation to medical science, and Ludwig Choulant's monumental *History and bibliography of anatomic illustration* (1945) is another example of attempts to survey the extensive subject of the illustration of medical subjects by artists. Lucien Hahn (1962) published a finely illustrated history of medical book illustration, based on the valuable collections housed in the Faculté de Médecine de Paris.

Egypt, India, China and Greece were the first countries to produce medical texts, and although those emanating from India were not illustrated, there were diagrammatic representations in those from China. In Egypt there were medical schools at an early date, notably at Alexandria and Edfu, and the practice of mummification ensured some knowledge of anatomy. Disease and deformities were recognised, and ancient papyri devoted to medical subjects include the Kahun Medical Papyrus written about 2100 B.C., the Edwin Smith Papyrus dating from about 1600 B.C., and the Papyrus Ebers and the Hearst Medical Papyrus, both written about 1550 B.C. These and several others have been studied and translated, further information on these translations being available in Thornton (1966, pp. 2–4). Carole Reeves (1980) has provided information on illustrations of medicine in ancient Egypt, including information on illustrations of medicine in ancient Egypt, including photographs of wall-carvings, stone slabs and statuettes, as well as an Ancient Egyptian birth scene, which is diagrammatic, with the child's head and limbs like those of an adult and so very large compared with the figure of the woman giving birth.

After the invention of printing in the middle of the fifteenth century, diagrams and other illustrations soon began to appear in medical and scientific books. These were woodcuts and wood engravings, which were then displaced by copper engravings, although wood was again employed at a later date. Although a number of books published on the Continent were well illustrated, few medical books published in England before the eighteenth century were outstanding for their plates. Furthermore, little is known of the artists responsible for the original drawings, a notable exception being the illustrations to *De fabrica* written by Andreas Vesalius (1514–1564) and published in Basle in 1543 and 1555. The drawings by Johann Stephan van Calcar (died 1546) were copied extensively in later publications, including *Compendiosa totius anatomice delineatio,* printed in London in 1545 with copper engravings by Thomas Geminus (died 1562). This is said to be the first illustrated textbook of anatomy published in England, and the copper plates the first to be engraved there.

Those depicting medical subjects were sometimes the authors of the texts, but were usually artists by profession, normally engaged in engraving copies of outstanding paintings. None could be identified as a specialised medical artist, devoting most of his life to drawing dissections so accurately that they might survive as outstanding examples in the history of medical art.

Jan Van Rymsdyk would probably have been astonished if anybody had suggested that his medical illustrations would survive for two centuries, and that his name would endure in the history of medical art as that of one of its most influential exponents. His birth and death remain shrouded in obscurity, and no personal diaries, letters, portraits or belongings have been found to throw any light on his activities. His *Museum Britannicum* contains information which enables us to appreciate his aspirations, his personal animosities, and to reconstruct the part of his character which was probably clouded by a sense of failure to achieve his ambition.

Rymsdyk had hoped to make a living, if not to achieve fame, as a portrait painter, and appears to have harboured a grievance against William Hunter for not helping him in this project. Rymsdyk did attempt to break away from medical illustration by leaving London and settling in Bristol. He advertised himself as a painter or portraits, and actually gained some commissions, but the few surviving portraits attributed to him from this period are neither signed nor dated. In fact, although traditionally the artist was said to be Rymsdyk, at one time they were thought to have been by his son Andrew which, for various reasons, was not possible.

Although Jan Van Rymsdyk's name appears on many of his drawings and engravings, he seldom received adequate recognition from his patrons. Some prefaces record his contributions as the artist responsible for the plates, but William Hunter, for whom most of Rymsdyk's drawings were executed, did not even name him in the preface to the *Gravid uterus*, although Robert Strange, who engraved two of the plates, is given fulsome praise. They are indeed, remarkable examples of the engraver's art, but it must also be recognised that their value lies in the fact that they are exact reproductions of the original drawings by Rymsdyk. William Hunter appreciated the skill of Rymsdyk to the extent of employing his services over a period of twenty years, not only for all but three of the plates in the *Gravid uterus*, but for many other subjects. All these drawings were carefully preserved, and when William Smellie's effects were eventually sold, William Hunter purchased Rymsdyk's original drawings for Smellie's atlas. They are now in the Hunterian Collection at Glasgow.

When historians records the virtues of the great anatomical and obstetrical atlases of the eighteenth century, they are usually associated with the names of their authors, William Smellie, William Hunter and possibly C. N. Jenty and Thomas Denman, although the publications of the two latter are more rare, and only to be found in the larger medical libraries. Yet the real value of these books is in their plates, and the artist initially responsible for most of these was Jan Van Rymsdyk. Even in books on medical illustration, in reference books containing the names of artists and engravers, and in collective biographies, his name may be mentioned with only the briefest details (generally inaccurate), because we know so little about Rymsdyk the man. Recognition of his work as an artist can only come second-hand through the engraved versions of his drawings, and from the originals preserved at Glasgow, the Royal College of Surgeons of England, the British Museum, and in Pennsylvania Hospital.

The illustrations in the atlases of both Smellie and William Hunter were flagrantly plagiarised on many occasions well into the nineteenth century. Seldom was their original source acknowledged, and they were always reduced in size and re-engraved, suffering much in the process. Plagiarism has been rife in publishing since the invention of printing, and many important texts have appeared with various imprints, within the space of a few years. William Harvey's *De generatione,* for example, was issued in 1651 by four different publishers, one in London and three in Amsterdam. Books with outstanding illustrations suffered even worse, sets of the plates being obtained by unscrupulous authors and published with their own texts, with no acknowledgement of the original source of the engravings.

Authors were those initially responsible for the publication of books. They usually paid the artists and engravers, supplied the captions and the text, and sometimes even paid for, or contributed towards, the cost of printing. Surely they were entitled to credit for the resultant work; they would inevitably suffer for defects in any of the processes involved. The artisans were employed to practise their respective crafts, and were paid accordingly. They were not regarded as members of separate professions, such as medicine and the law, until they organised themselves to form associations with rules and regulations, and examinations before admittance to membership. A system evolved similar to that of trade unions, and brought with it professional recognition. Even before this, printers, for example, became noted for the quality of their work, taking pride in the type faces, paper and ink involved in producing beautiful books. John Baskerville was an outstanding example, and William Hunter chose him to print his *Gravid uterus*. But he gave scant credit to the artist employed by him on a long-term basis to make drawings, although it was he who really made the book endure as the outstanding atlas of that and succeeding centuries.

The mezzotint and copper engravings of Jan Van Rymsdyk's original drawings were extensively used for teaching purposes, and the individual plates were framed and displayed in dissecting rooms and lecture theatres. The high cost of producing folio atlases has always deterred their acquisition by the majority of students, but their value in medical education has been widely appreciated. Lecturers have used diagrams and drawings to illustrate their talks, particulary when demonstration from actual specimens was difficult or impossible, and although plaster casts and museum specimens have largely been displaced by audio-visual aids, illustrated books have not yet been entirely displaced by tapes, television and other mechanical aids. There is still the need for lecturers to answer queries, to up-date words recorded in the past, and for medical artists to depict features not readily recordable by the camera. Artists would find inspiration in the work of Rymsdyk, who achieved remarkable results without the aid of modern techniques, working against time to record the minute details of rapidly decaying dissection subjects.

The Rymsdyk drawings from dissections by Jenty, still preserved in the Pennsylvania Hospital, played an important part in early medical education in the United States, and students of medicine and of art can still profit from viewing his drawings or the engraved versions published in books by Hunter, Smellie and Denman. These are available in most large medical libraries, and are still worth studying as worthy reproductions of conditions which have not undergone any significant changes since they were drawn.

Medical artists have only recently been formed into a professional body, and their services to medical science in general, and medical education in particular, are beginning to be appreciated. They form an important branch of the medical auxiliaries providing the main support for the medical profession. They should study the history of medical illustration, and evaluate the work of their predecessors. Supreme among these would inevitably be Jan Van Rymsdyk, whose original drawings exist as proof of his monumental contributions as interpreted by the engravers, and who might well be adopted as the patron saint of medical artists, and as the father of British medical illustration.

BIBLIOGRAPHY

This contains the references used in the preparation of this book, most of which are noted in the text by the name of the author followed by the date of publication in parentheses. Additional material can be traced by reference to the Wellcome Institute for the History of Medicine *Subject catalogue of the history of medicine and related sciences*, 17 vols., Munich, *Kraus*, 1980, and to *Current Work in the History of Medicine.*

Allan, D.G.C. (1974). *The houses of the Royal Society of Arts: a history and a guide. (Second, revised edition).* London, *Royal Society of Arts,* 1974.

Anderson, William (1885). An outline of the history of art in its relation to medical science. *St. Thomas's Hospital Reports*, 15, 1885, pp. 151-181.

Asherson, N. (1979). David Bayford, his syndrome and sign of dysphagia lusoria. *Annals of the Royal College of Surgeons of England*, 61, 1979, pp. 63-67.

Barbour, A.H.F. (1888). *Early contributions of anatomy to obstetrics. . . . Read before the Edinburgh Obstetrical Society, 9th May, 1888.* Edinburgh, 1888.

Brock, Helen (1974). James Douglas of the pouch. *Medical History*, 18, 1974, pp. 162 - 172.

Bunch, Antonia J. (1975). *Hospital and medical libraries in Scotland. An historical and sociological study.* Glasgow, *Scottish Library Association,* 1975.

Cameron, S.J. (1957). William Smellie. *Scottish Medical Journal*, 2, 1957, pp. 439 - 444.

Camper, Pieter (Petrus) (1939). Itera in Angliam 1748 - 1785. *Opuscula Selecta Neerlandicorum de Arte Medica*, 15, 1939.

Choulant, Ludwig (1945). *History and bibliography of anatomic illustration. . . . Translated and annotated by Mortimer Frank. Further essays by Fielding H. Garrison, Mortimer Frank, Edward C. Streeter, with a new historical essay by Charles Singer, and a bibliography of Mortimer Frank by J. Christian Bay.* New York, London, *Hafner,* 1945, (reprinted 1962).

Corner, Betsy Copping (1951). Dr. Ibis and the artists: a sidelight upon Hunter's atlas, The gravid uterus. *Journal of the History of Medicine*, 6, 1951, pp. 1 - 21.

De Lint, J.G. (1916). The plates of Jenty. *Janus*, 21, 1916, pp. 129 - 135.

Dobson, Jessie (1951). The Hunter specimens at Kew Observatory. *Annals of the Royal College of Surgeons of England*, 8, 1951, pp. 457 - 462.

Dobson, Jessie (1954). The Army Nursing Service in the eighteenth century. *Annals of the Royal College of Surgeons of England*, 14, 1954, pp. 417 - 419.

Dobson, Jessie (1969). John Hunter's artists. *Medical and Biological Illustration*, 9, 1959, pp. 138 - 149.

Dobson, Jessie (1959). *John Hunter.* Edinburgh, London, *Livingstone*, 1969.

Dobson, Jessie (1970). *Descriptive catalogue of the Physiological Series in the Hunterian Museum of the Royal College of Surgeons of England. Part 1. Surviving specimens demonstrating these organs in plants and animals for the special purpose of the individual.* Edinburgh, London, *Livingstone*, 1970.

Dossie, Robert (1782). *Memoirs of agriculture, and other oeconomical arts.* Vol. 3, London, *for C. Nourse*, 1782.

Edwards, Edward (1808). *Anecdotes of painters who have resided or been born in England*, London, *Leigh & Sotheby*, 1808.

Foskett, Daphne (1972). *A dictionary of British miniature painters.* London, *Faber*, 1972.

Fothergill, John (1971). *Chain of friendship. Selected letters of Dr. John Fothergill of London, 1735 - 1780. With introduction and notes by Betsy C. Corner & Christopher C. Booth.* Cambridge, Mass., *Harvard University Press*, 1971.

Fox, R. Hingston (1901). *William Hunter, anatomist, physician, obstetrician, (1718 - 1783), with notices of his friends Cullen, Smellie, Fothergill, and Baillie.* London, *H.K. Lewis*, 1901.

Gask, George E. (1936 - 37). John Hunter in the campaign in Portugal, 1762 - 1763. *British Journal of Surgery*, 24, 1936 - 37, pp. 640 - 668. (Also in his *Essays in the history of medicine*, London, *Butterworth*, 1950, pp. 116 - 144).

George, M. Dorothy (1979). *London life in the eighteenth century.* Harmondsworth, Mddx., *Penguin Books*, 1979. (First published 1925).

Glaister, John (1894). *Dr. William Smellie and his contempories. A contribution to the history of midwifery in the eighteenth century.* Glasgow, *James MacLehose*, 1894.

Gloyne, S. Roodhouse (1950). *John Hunter.* Edinburgh, *Livingstone*, 1950.

Goodall, A. L. (1958). The writings of William Hunter. *The Bibliotheck*, 1, iv, 1958, pp. 46 - 47.

Graves, Algernon (1906). *The Royal Academy of Arts. A complete dictionary of contributors and their work from its foundation in 1769 to 1904.* Vol. 5, London, *Henry Graves & George Bell*, 1906. (Republished by S.R. Publishers and Kingsmead Reprints, 1970, Vol. 3 comprising Vols. 5 & 6 of the original).

Graves, Algernon (1907). *The Society of Artists of Great Britain 1760 - 1791. The Free Society of Artists 1761 - 1783. A complete dictionary of contributors and their work from the foundation of the Societies to 1791.* Bath, *Kingsmead Reprints,* 1969. (First published 1907).

Greim, Florence M. (1952). Anatomical illustrations from the Fothergill Collection at the Pennsylvania Hospital, with a foreword by Florence M. Greim. *What's New*, April, 1952.

Gunn, Alistair L. (1967 - 68). The inevitable William and the accidental John. (Hunterian Oration, 1968). *Transactions of the Hunterian Society,* 1967-68, pp. 87 - 103.

Hahn, André, *et al.* (1962). *Histoire de la médecine et du livre médical, a la lumière des collections de la Bibliothèque de la Faculté de Médicine de Paris. André Hahn, Paule Dumaitre, avec la collaboration de Janine Samion-Contet.* Paris, *Olivier Perrin*, 1962.

Hudson, Derek, and Luckhurst, Kenneth W. (1954). *The Royal Society of Arts, 1754 - 1954, (etc.).* London, *John Murray*, 1954.

Huffman, John W. (1969). Jan Van Rymsdyk, medical illustrator extraordinary. *Journal of the American Medical Association,* 208,1969, pp. 121 - 124.

Huffman, John W. (1970). The great eighteenth century obstetric atlases and their illustrator. *Obstetrics and Gynecology*, 35, 1970, pp. 971 - 976.

Illingworth, *Sir* Charles (1971). William Hunter's manuscripts and letters: the Glasgow Collection. *Medical History*, 15, 1971, pp. 181 - 186.

Johnstone, R. W. (1952). *William Smellie: the master of British midwifery.* Edinburgh, London, *Livingstone*, 1952.

Kemp, Martin (1975). *Dr. William Hunter at the Royal Academy of Arts. Edited by Martin Kemp.* Glasgow, *University of Glasgow Press*, 1975.

Kemp, Martin (1976). Dr. William Hunter and the Windsor Leonardos, and his volume of drawings attributed to Pietro da Cortona. *Burlington Magazine*, 118, 1976, pp. 144 - 148.

Krivatsy, Peter (1968). Le Blon's anatomical color engravings. *Journal of the History of Medicine*, 23, 1968, pp. 153 - 158.

Krumbhaar, E. B. (1922). The early history of anatomy in the United States. *Annals of Medical History,* 4, 1922, pp. 271 - 286.

LeFanu, William R. (1946). *John Hunter: a list of his books.* London, *Royal College of Surgeons of England*, 1946.

LeFanu, William R. (1958). The writings of William Hunter, F.R.S. *The Bibliotheck*, 1, iii, 1958, pp. 3 - 14.

LeFanu, William R. (1978). Natural history drawings collected by John Hunter, F.R.S. (1728 - 1793), at the Royal College of Surgeons of England. *Journal of the Society for the Bibliography of Natural History*, 8, 1978, pp. 329 - 333.

Little, Bryan (1980). *Bath portrait. The story of Bath, its life and its buildings. (4th edition).* Bristol, *Burleigh Press*, 1980.

Long, Basil (1929). *British miniaturists.* London, *Bles*, 1929.

Marks, Arthur S. (1967). An anatomical drawing by Alexander Cozens. *Journal of the Warburg and Courtauld Institutes*, 30, 1967, pp. 434 - 438.

Ollerenshaw, R. (1974). Dr. Hunter's 'Gravid uterus' - a bicentenary note. *Medical and Biological Illustration*, 24, 1974, pp. 43 - 57.

Oppenheimer, Jane M. (1946). *New aspects of John and William Hunter. I. Everard Home and the destruction of the John Hunter manuscripts. II. William Hunter and his contemporaries.* New York, *Schuman*, 1946.

Packard, F. R. (1938). *Some account of the Pennsylvania Hospital from its rise to the beginning of the year 1938.* Philadelphia, *Pennsylvania Hospital*, 1938.

Peachey, George C. (1924). *A memoir of William & John Hunter.* Plymouth, *Wm. Brendon, for the author*, 1924.

Peachey, George C. (1930). William Hunter's obstetrical career. *Annals of Medical History*, N.S.2, 1930, pp. 476 - 479.

Redgrave, S. (1878). *A dictionary of artists of the English School.* London, 1878.

Reeves, Carole (1980). Illustrations of medicine in Ancient Egypt. *Journal of Audiovisual Media in Medicine*, 3, 1980, pp. 4 - 13.

Robb-Smith, A. H. T. (1970). John Hunter's private press. *Journal of the History of Medicine*, 25, 1970, pp. 262 - 269.

Royal Society of Arts. Minutes of Committees 1766 - 7. (MS.)

Russell, K. F. (1963). *British anatomy 1525 - 1800: a bibliography.* Melbourne, *Melbourne University Press*, 1963.

Schumann, Edward A. (1940 - 41). William Hunter lecturing on obstetrics and infant care. *Transactions and Studies of the College of Physicians of Philadelphia*, 4th series, 8, 1940 - 41, pp. 155 - 183.

Scott, J. A. (1904). Concerning the Fothergill pictures at the Pennsylvania Hospital. *University of Pennsylvania Medical Bulletin*, 16, 1904, pp. 388 - 393.

Scott, Joseph C., Hunt, Arthur B., and Keys, Thomas E. (1964). A note on William Hunter's monograph *The anatomy of the human gravid uterus. Mayo Clinic Proceedings*, 39, 1964, pp. 197 - 204.

Smith, Brian S., and Ralph, Elizabeth (1972). *A history of Bristol and Gloucestershire.* Beaconsfield, *Darwen Finlayson*, 1972.

Smith, G. Munro (1917). *A history of the Bristol Royal Infirmary.* Bristol, *Arrowsmith*; London, *Simpkin Marshall*, 1917.

Smith, Richard. Bristol Infirmary Biographical Memoirs, 1735 - 77, (14 volumes), Vol. 2, (MS. and cuttings).

Spencer, Herbert R. (1927). *The history of British midwifery from 1650 - 1800. Fitz-Patrick Lectures for 1927 delivered before the Royal College of Physicians of London*, London, *Bale & Danielson*, 1927.

Stark, J. Nigel (1908). *An obstetric diary of William Hunter, 1762 - 1765. Edited, with notes, by J. Nigel Stark. Reprinted from the "Glasgow Medical Journal".* Glasgow, *printed by Alex Macdougall*, 1908.

Summerson, *Sir* John (1778). *Georgian London.* Harmondsworth, Mdax., *Penguin Books,* 1978.

Tait, Haldane P., and Wallace, Archibald T. (1952). Dr. William Smellie and his Library at Lanark, Scotland. *Bulletin of the History of Medicine,* 26, 1952, pp. 403 - 421.

Teacher, John H. (1900). *Catalogue of the anatomical and pathological preparations of Dr. William Hunter in the Hunterian Museum, University of Glasgow.* 2 vols., Glasgow, *James MacLehose,* 1900.

Teacher, John H. (1970). *Catalogue of the anatomical preparations of Dr. William Hunter in the Museum of the Anatomy Department, compiled by Alice J. Marshall from the original catalogue (1899 - 1900) prepared by John Teacher.* Glasgow, *University of Glasgow,* 1970.

Thomas, K. Bryn (1960). A female foetus, drawn from nature by Mr. Blakey for William Hunter. *Medical History,* 4, 1960, p. 256.

Thomas, K. Bryn (1964). *James Douglas of the pouch, and his pupil William Hunter.* London, *Pitman,* 1964.

Thomas, K. Bryn (1974). The great anatomical atlases. *Proceedings of the Royal Society of Medicine,* 67, 1974, pp. 223 - 232.

Thomson, John (1859). *An account of the life, lectures, and writings of William Cullen,* 2 vols., Edinburgh, London, *Blackwood,* 1859.

Thornton, John L. (1966). *Medical books, libraries and collectors: a study of bibliography and the book trade in relation to medical science. 2nd edition.* London, *Deutsch,* 1966.

Thornton, John L., and Tully, R. I. J. (1971). *Scientific books, libraries and collectors: a study of bibliography and the book trade in relation to science. 3rd edition.* London, *Library Association,* 1971. *Supplement, 1969 -*

1975, 1978.

Thornton, John L., and Want, Patricia C. (1974a). Artist versus engraver in William Hunter's "Anatomy of the human gravid uterus", 1774. *Medical and Biological Illustration,* 24, 1974, pp. 137 - 139.

Thornton, John L., and Want, Patricia C. (1974b). William Hunter's "The anatomy of the human gravid uterus", 1774 - 1974. *Journal of Obstetrics and Gynaecology of the British Commonwealth,* 81, 1974, pp. 1 - 10.

Thornton, John L., and Want, Patricia C. (1978). Charles Nicholas Jenty and the mezzotint plates in his "Demonstrations of a pregnant uterus", 1757. *Journal of Audiovisual Media in Medicine,* 1, 1978, pp. 113 - 115.

Thornton, John L., and Want, Patricia C. (1979). Jan Van Rymsdyk's illustrations of the gravid uterus drawn for Hunter, Smellie, Jenty and Denman. *Journal of Audiovisual Media in Medicine,* 2, 1979, pp. 10 - 15.

INDEX

A

Abortions, 38
Adam's Weekly Courant, 80
Albinus, Bernhard Siegfried, 26, 57
Alfreton Park, Derbyshire, 80, 81
Aliamet, François, 31, 35
Alison, David, 12
Allan, D. G. C., 75; *bib.*, 94
Allen, "Thumbs", portrait by Rymsdyk, 6, 7
Amsterdam, Rymsdyk in, 2
Anatomical description of the human gravid uterus (William Hunter), 31
Anatomy of the human gravid uterus (William Hunter), 27 - 40
    drawings by Rymsdyk at Glasgow, 31
Anderson, William, 89; *bib.*, 94
Animals, group painted by Rymsdyk, 49
Aristotle, 25
Artists, medical, 90, 92 - 3
Asbestos, 2
Aselli, Gasparo, 57
Asherson, N., 87, *bib.*, 94
Athlone, *Earl of,* 81
Aubrey, Mary, 81
Auckland University, 21

B

Baillie, Matthew, 31, 41, 82, 83 - 4
Barbour, A. H. F., 25; *bib.*, 94

Barrett, William, 6, 7
    portrait by Rymsdyk, 7 - 8
Baskerville, John, 28 - 9, 39, 92
Bath, Andrew Van Rymsdyk at, 79 - 81
    Victoria Art Gallery, 80
Bath Chronicle, 79, 80, 81
Bath Literary Club, 80
Bay, J. Christian, *bib.*, 94
Bayford, David, 87
Behn, *Mrs.* A., 65
Bell, William, 45
Belle Isle, 44, 54
Berengario da Carpi, Giacomo, 26
Bibliotheca Walleriana, 55
Blakey, Nicholas, 35
Book illustration, medical, Rymsdyk's influence on, 89 - 93
Bower, Alban, 80
Bower, Janet M., 80 - 1
Boyle, Peter, 9, 61, 67 - 9
Bristol, in eighteenth century, 5 - 6
    Rymsdyk in, 2 - 3, 5 - 7
Bristol Museum and Art Gallery, 6, 7
Bristol Royal Infirmary, 6
British Museum, 41, 61 - 2, *et seq.*
    Dept. of Prints and Drawings, Rymsdyk drawings in, 69 - 74, 87
Brock, Helen, 24, 39, 40; *bib.*, 94
Brodie, Elizabeth, 83
Bryer, Henry, 32, 35
Buffalo, head drawn by Rymsdyk, 87
Bunch, Antonia J., 12, *bib.*, 94
Burgess, Thomas, 58, 60
Burt, G. M., 16
Burton, John, 11

C

Calcar, Johann Stephan van, 90
Cameron, S. J., 11; *bib.*, 94
Camper, Pieter, 15 - 7; *bib.*, 94

Canot, Charles, 35
Cant, Arent, 57
Case, Henry, 81
Charlotte, *Queen*, 24, 49, 66 - 7
Charpentier, 58
Chereau, 58
Cheselden, William, 3, 44
Chester, Andrew Van Rymsdyk in, 80
Chick, development, drawn by Rymsdyk, 49 - 51, 66, 71 - 2
Childbirth, 27
Choulant, Ludwig, 89; *bib.*, 94; *quoted*, 22
Clark, John, 84
Clift, William, 45, 49, 52, 66 - 7
Coker, Mary Aubrey, 81
Collection of engravings (Denman), Rymsdyk's drawings for, 84 - 7
Coloured copperplates, 57
    mezzotints, 55, 57
    woodcuts, 57
Company of Surgeons, 58, 60
Cooper, *Dr.*, 83
Copperplates, coloured, 57
Cornelius, Eustace H., 43
Corner, Betsy Copping, 64; *bib.*, 95
Cozens, Alexander, 35
Croft, *Sir* Richard, 83 - 4
Cruikshank, William, 41
Cullen, William, 23
    letters from William Hunter, 30 - 1

D

Danzel, 58
Dartmouth, *Earl of*, 62
De Lint, J. G., 54; *bib.*, 95
Demonstrations of a pregnant uterus (Jenty), Rymsdyk's drawings for, 54 - 5, 57 - 60
Denman, John, 82 - 3
Denman, Joseph, 83

Denman, Thomas, 20, 39
  biographical, 82 - 4
  Rymsdyk's drawings for, 9, 82 - 8
Denman, Thomas, *Lord Chief Justice*, 84
Dobson, Jessie, 43, 45, 49, 54, 67; *bib.*, 95
Dossie, Robert, 75; *bib.*, 95
Douglas, James, 23 - 4
Douglas, Martha Jane, 23
Douglas, William, 11
Douglas, William George, 23, 24
Draper, *Mrs.*, 24
Dumaitre, Paule, *bib.*, 26

E
Earl's Court, 44
Edinburgh University, 12
Edkins, Michael, 6, 7
Edkins, William, 7
Edwards, Edward, 32, 81; *bib.*, 95
Egg, hen's, development, drawn by Rymsdyk, 49 - 51
Eggs, birds', drawn by the Rymsdyks, 71 - 2
Egypt, ancient, medical illustrations in, 89 - 90
Embryology, early studies of, 25 - 6
  of chick, Rymsdyk's drawings of, 49 - 51, 66
Engravers, Rymsdyk on, 62, 64
Engravings, representing the generation of some animals (Denman), Rymsdyk's drawings in, 85 - 7
Essay on the demonstration of the human structure (Jenty), Rymsdyk's drawings for, 54 - 6
Eustachius, Bartholomaeus, 26

F
Fallopius, Gabriel, 26
Felix Farley's Bristol Journal, 6
Fisher, Edward, 55, 58
Forceps, obstetric, 11, 20 - 1

Foskett, Daphne, 80; *bib.*, 95
Fothergill, John, 58, 60, 69; *bib.*, 95
Fox, R. Hingston, 22; *bib.*, 95
Frank, Mortimer, *bib.*, 94
Frye, Thomas, 2 - 3

G
Galen, 25
Garthshore, M., 87
Gask, George E., 54; *bib.*, 95
Gautier d'Agoty, Jacques Fabian, 57
Geminus, Thomas, 90
General Evening Post, 20
George III, 49, 66
George, M. Dorothy, 3; *bib.*, 95
Gillard, Joe, 7
Gilmour, Ruth G., 81
Glaister, John, 12, 21; *bib.*, 95
Glasgow University, Hunterian Collection, 20, 22, 33, 40, 41, 91
Gloyne, S. Roodhouse, 43; *bib.*, 95
Goodall, A. L., 25; *bib.*, 96
Graaf, Regnier de, 26
Graves, Algernon, 76 - 7; *bib.*, 96
Great Windmill Street School of Anatomy, 24, 41
Greim, Florence M., 60; *bib.*, 96; *quoted*, 53
Grignion, Charles, 12, 15, 17, 20, 32, 45, 48
    engraving of Smellie portrait, 13
Gunn, Alistair L., 22; *bib.*, 96; *quoted*, 10

H
Hague, The, Rymsdyk in, 2
Hahn, André, 89; *bib.*, 96
Haighton, John, 39 - 40
Haller, Albrecht von, 26
Hamilton, *Sir* William, 69, 73
Harvey, William, 91

Harvie, *Dr.* John, 11, 20
Harvie, John, Writer to the Signet, 12
Hen's egg, development, drawn by Rymsdyk, 49 - 51
Hippocrates, 25
Holland, Rymsdyk's early life in, 1 - 2
Home, *Sir* Everard, 44, 49, 52
Hudson, Derek, 75; *bib.*, 96
Huffman, John W., 1; *bib.*, 96
Hunt, Arthur B., 40; *bib.*, 97 - 8
Hunter, James, 23
Hunter, John, 4, 7 - 9, 23, 27, 29 - 30, 41, 42
    biographical, 43 - 5
    Rymsdyk's drawings for, 5, 43 - 52
    specimens given to Kew Observatory, 66 - 7
Hunter, William, 11, 27
    biographical, 23 - 5
    letters to William Cullen, 30 - 1
    purchase of Rymsdyk's drawings for Smellie, 20
    Rymsdyk's attack on "Doctor Ibis", 64 - 6
    Rymsdyk's drawings for, 4, 9, 17, 22 - 42
Hunterian Collection, Glasgow University, 20, 22, 33, 40, 41, 91

I

"Ibis, Dr.", attacked by Rymsdyk, 64 - 6
Illingworth, *Sir* Charles, 22, 39; *bib.*, 96
Illustration, medical, history of, 89 - 90
    medical book, Rymsdyk's influence on, 89 - 93
Introduction to the practice of midwifery (Denman), Rymsdyk's drawings in, 85

J

Jamaica, possible visit by Rymsdyk, 74
Jenner, Edward, 43, 44, 45
Jenty, Charles Nicholas, 7 - 9, 27
    Rymsdyk's drawings for, 5, 53 - 60
Johnson, J., 52
Johnstone, R. W., 10, 12, 16, 21; *bib.*, 96
Jordaens, Jacob, 9

K
Kemp, Martin, 25, 26; *bib.*, 96
Kew Observatory, 49, 66 - 7
Keys, Thomas E., 40; *bib.*, 97 - 8
King's College, London, 49, 66 - 7
Kleinfeldt, *Miss* D. M., 80
Krivatsy, Peter, 59; *bib.*, 96
Krohn, Henry, 83
Krumbhaar, E. B., 58 - 9, *bib.*, 96

L
Ladmiral, Jan, 57
Lanark, Grammar School, 11 - 12
    Lindsay Institute, 11 - 12
Lancisi, Giovanni, 26
Le Blon, Jacob Christoph, 57
LeFanu, William R., 25, 48, 52; *bib.*, 97; *quoted*, 43
Leonardo da Vinci, 25 - 6
Leyden University, Camper drawings in, 16
Lindsay Institute, Lanark, 11 - 12
Little, Bryan, 79; *bib.*, 97
London, in eighteenth century, 3 - 4
    Rymsdyk's arrival in, 4
London Evening Post, 11
Long, Basil, *bib.*, 97
Longfellow, Henry Wadsworth, *quoted*, 89
Luckhurst, Kenneth W., 75; *bib.*, 96
Lumley, Edward, 40
Lyne, Edward, portrait by Rymsdyk, 6

M
Maas, Karina, 7
Macaulay, George, 87
McClintock, Alfred H., 12, 14
Major, Thomas, 31

Maleuvre, Pierre, 32
Marks, Arthur S., 35; *bib.*, 97
Marshall, Alice J., 22; *bib.*, 98
Martin, Elias, 62, 64
Martin, Frederick, 62, 64
Mechel, 32
Medical artists, 90, 92 - 3
Medical book illustration, Rymsdyk's influence on, 89 - 93
Medical Observations and Inquiries, 40, 87
Menil, 35, 38
Mezzotint, use in Jenty's atlases, 55 - 8
Midwives, male, 27
Miller, J., 40
Miniatures, painted by Andrew Van Rymsdyk, 79 - 81
Mitchel, J., 32
Mondino de' Luzzi (Mundinus), 25
Monro, Alexander (1697 - 1767), 23
Moore, J., 62, 63
Morewood, Henry Case, 80 - 81
Muscio (or Moschion), 25
Museum Britannicum (Rymsdyk), 1 - 2, 9, 41 - 2, 61 - 74

N

National Gallery of Ireland, Dublin, miniatures by Andrew Van Rymsdyk in, 81
Natural history of the human teeth (John Hunter), Rymsdyk's drawings for, 44 - 5
Netherlands, Rymsdyk's early life in, 1 - 2
Newton, Thomas, *Bishop of Bristol*, portrait by Rymsdyk, 6
Nicholls, Frank, 11, 24
Nihell, *Mrs.*, 11
Norfolk Chronicle, 80
North, *Lord*, 62
Norwich, Andrew Van Rymsdyk in, 80

O

Observations on certain parts of the animal oeconomy (John Hunter), Rymsdyk drawings in, 45, 48
Ollerenshaw, R., 27; *bib.*, 97
Oppenheimer, Jane M., 52; *bib.*, 97
Osborn, *Lord*, 62
Osborn, William, 20
Ottley, Drewry, 49
Owen, *Sir* Richard, 52

P

Packard, F. R., 58, 60; *bib.*, 97
Page, John, portrait by Rymsdyk, 6
Page, Thomas, portrait by Frye, 2 - 3
Palmer, James F., 49
Peachey, George C., 22, 24, 43; *bib.*, 97
Peccary, in group of animals painted by Rymsdyk, 49
Pemberton, James, 58
Pembroke, Mary, *Countess of*, 80, 81
Pennsylvania Hospital, Rymsdyk drawings in, 54, 58 - 60, 92
Phillips, Miles, 11 - 2
Philosophical Transactions, 41, 45, 48
Portrait painter, Rymsdyk as, 5 - 7
Pott, Percivall, 44
Powle, 38
Purcell, Richard, 58

R

Rains, A. J. Harding, 43
Ralph, Elizabeth, 6; *bib.*, 98
Redgrave, S., *bib.*, 97
Reeves, Carole, 89 - 90; *bib.*, 97
Remsdyk, spellings of name, 1
Rhodes, Martha, 41

Richardson, John, 52
Riemsdyk, spellings of name, 1
Rigby, Edward, 31
Robb-Smith, A. H. T., 52; *bib.*, 97
Roederer, Johann Georg, 26
Royal Academy of Arts, 24 - 5, 62, 77, 80
Royal College of Physicians of Edinburgh, Camper drawings in, 16
Royal College of Physicians of London, 12
Royal College of Obstetricians and Gynaecologists, 12
Royal College of Surgeons of Edinburgh, portrait of Smellie in, 12
Royal College of Surgeons of England, 39
John Hunter specimens from Kew in, 66 - 7
Rymsdyk drawings in, 43, 45, 48, 49 - 52
Royal Society of Arts, 75
Russell, K. F., 54; *bib.*, 97
Ruysch, Fredrik, 57
Ryland, 45
Rymsdyk, spellings of name, 1
Rymsdyk, Andrew Van, 1, 4, 7, 9, 75 - 81
drawings for *Museum Britannicum*, 64, 70, 72, 77 - 9
Rymsdyk, Van, (father of Jan), 2

S

St. Aubin, J., 45
Samion-Contet, Janine, *bib.*, 96
Sandwich, *Lord*, 74, 78
Scheveling, Rymsdyk in, 2
Schumann, Edward A., 39; *bib.*, 97
Scotin, Louis Gerard, 31
Scott, J. A., 58; *bib.*, 97
Scott, Joseph C., 40; *bib.*, 97 - 8
Seligman, J. M., 58
Sett of anatomical tables (Smellie), Camper's drawings for, 15 - 7
Rymsdyk's drawings for, 14 - 21
Sewell, Jem, 7
Shelley, P. B., *quoted*, 75
"Ship, The" tavern in Bristol, 7

Shippen, William, 58, 60
Siddons, *Mrs.*, 81
Sign-painter, Rymsdyk as, 7
Singer, Charles, *bib.*, 94
Sloane, *Sir* Hans, 69, 74, 78
Smellie, John, 12
Smellie, William, 3, 23, 27
    biographical, 10 - 2
    Rymsdyk's drawings for, 4 - 5, 10 - 21
    Rymsdyk's portrait of, 5, 12 - 3
    self-portrait, 12
Smith, Brian S., 6; *bib.*, 98
Smith, G. Munro, 6 - 7; *bib.*, 98
Smith, Richard, 2, 6, 7; *bib.*, 98
Smollett, Tobias, 11, 12
Society of Artists of Great Britain, 76 - 7
Solms, Frederick Henry, and Emilia Van, *Prince and Princess of Orange*, mezzotint by Rymsdyk, 9
Soranus of Ephesus, 25
Spencer, Herbert R., 82; *bib.*, 98
Sprague, Martha, 2
Stark, J. Nigel, 24; *bib.*, 98
St. Aubin, J., 45
Strange, *Sir* Robert, 30, 31 - 2, 34, 45
Streeter, Edward C., *bib.*, 94
Strong, William, 7
Summerson, *Sir* John, 3; *bib.*, 98
Sydenham Society, 40

T

Tait, Haldane P., 12; *bib.*, 98
Taylor, Henry, *quoted*, 1
Teacher, John H., 22, 41; *bib.*, 98
Teeth, Rymsdyk's drawings of, 45
Thicknesse, Philip, 11
Thomas, K. Bryn, 23 - 4, 35, 40; *bib.*, 98
Thomson, Henry, 41
Thomson, John, 23, 29 - 30; *bib.*, 98

Thornton, John L., 27, 54, 85, 89; *bib.*, 98 - 9
Tickell, Elizabeth Ann, 80
Tickell, *Mrs.* Richard, 80
Tully, R. I. J., *bib.*, 98 - 9
Tyson, William, 6

U

Uppsala University, Waller Library, 55
Uterus, gravid, early studies of, 25 - 7

V

Van Solms, Frederick Henry, and Emilia, *Prince and Princess of Orange*, mezzotint by Rymsdyk, 9
Vater, Abraham, 26
Vesalius, Andreas, 26, 90
Victoria and Albert Museum, miniatures by Andrew Van Rymsdyk in, 81
Victoria Art Gallery, Bath, miniature by Andrew Van Rymsdyk in, 80

W

Walker, William, 7
Wallace, Archibald T., 12; *bib.*, 98
Waller Library, Uppsala University, 55
Wandelaer, Jan, 26
Want, Patricia C., 27, 54, 85; *bib.*, 99
Wellcome Historical Medical Library, 69
White, Charles, 64
Wilkie, James, 24
Wolff, Caspar, 25
Woodcuts, coloured, 57
Worlidge, Thomas, 38